THE RECIPE FOR
Breastfeeding Support
IN AMERICA

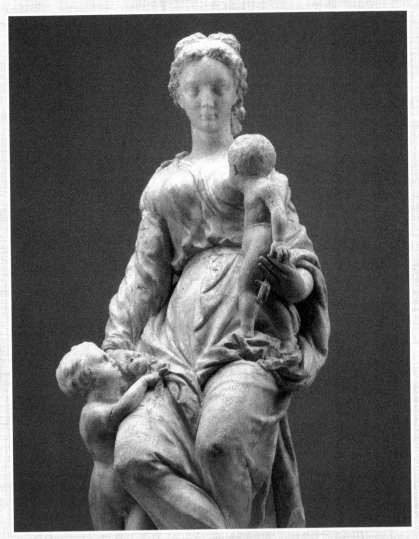

Jacques Du Broeucq, Netherlandish, circa 1505–1584; *Charity*, 16th century; alabaster; 24 x 11 13/16 x 7 1/16 inches; Saint Louis Art Museum, Museum Purchase 64:1928.

THE RECIPE FOR
Breastfeeding Support
IN AMERICA

Erin L. O'Reilly

First Printing: 2020

This book was edited, designed, laid out, proofread, and publicized by an Editwright team.
Visit editwright.com for more Editwright works.

Developmental editing by Andrew Doty
Copy editing by Karen L. Tucker
Cover photo by Gabriella Marks
Proofreading by Lisa Ashpole
Book design by Peggy Nehmen

Published by Healthy Nourishment, LLC
Saint Louis, Missouri

Erin L. O'Reilly shares her experiences and knowledge as a public speaker for classes, workshops, seminars, and special events. To contact the author about speaking at an event, visit ErinLOReilly.com.

Library of Congress Control Number: 2020921275

Paperback ISBN: 978-1-7344388-0-2
E-book ISBN: 978-1-7344388-1-9

BISAC Codes:
HEA044000   HEALTH & FITNESS / Breastfeeding
MED036000   MEDICAL / Health Policy
HEA028000   HEALTH & FITNESS / Health Care Issues

Lovingly dedicated to:

My son, Jesse, who made me a mother and inspired me to breastfeed

My husband, Jay, who supported me to breastfeed in so many ways

My sister, Patricia, who helped me get through my difficulties

The seven La Leche League founders who started the mother-to-mother breastfeeding support group that I received so much inspiration and help from and who to this day have not received the recognition and accolades they deserve

WIC, the organization I worked for and, although I critique, I appreciate

All the breastfeeding mothers and babies I have worked with over the years

Contents

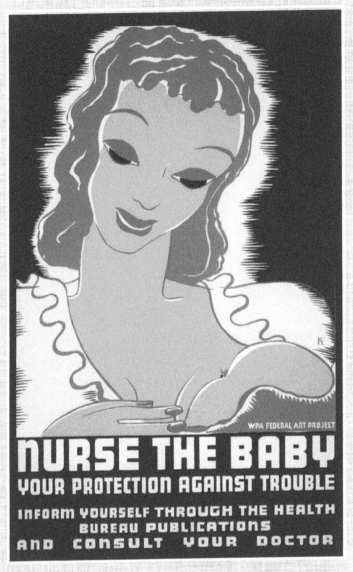

WPA FEDERAL ART PROJECT

NURSE THE BABY
YOUR PROTECTION AGAINST TROUBLE
INFORM YOURSELF THROUGH THE HEALTH BUREAU PUBLICATIONS
AND CONSULT YOUR DOCTOR

This US government poster was published in 1938 as part of the Works Progress Administration Federal Art Project to promote breastfeeding for public health. Our country wants us to breastfeed, but it doesn't even recognize our work to breastfeed and doesn't give us the support we need. This book is about what the US needs to do to support mothers to successfully breastfeed our babies!

Introduction

This book is about what "ingredients" are needed to effectively support breastfeeding mothers and babies. It is for everyone who has anything to do with mothers and babies, because *everyone* should support breastfeeding.

I am an International Board Certified Lactation Consultant (IBCLC) and a nurse with a background in public health nursing. Since the early 1980s, I've worked with moms and babies in many settings and situations: prenatal, labor and delivery, postnatal, the hospital, a community health care clinic, a WIC center, home visits with families, and volunteer community support. I am a La Leche League Leader, a WIC Breastfeeding Coordinator, and past president and current member of breastfeeding coalition(s). I work with moms of many cultures, colors, and nationalities. I've worked with younger, older, richer, poorer, gay, straight, well-educated, less-educated, exclusively and partially breastfeeding, expressed (pumped-milk) feeding, and even adoptive breastfeeding moms. I am also a mother myself; I breastfed my son and experienced firsthand many challenges and rewards of breastfeeding!

I enjoy my work and find it rewarding, but I am saddened and angered by the fact that America wants and expects mothers to breastfeed but refuses to give them the adequate support they need to be successful. My years of well-rounded experience, education, and training have qualified me to write this book about how America can and needs to give much greater recognition and support to breastfeeding moms and babies.

This is not a "how to breastfeed" book; rather, this is a "how to support breastfeeding mothers" book. This "recipe" for breastfeeding support will be broad in scope, and I will discuss the ingredients needed for breastfeeding support and success in America. I will elucidate many of the systemic, medical, legal, policy, economic, and social issues that exist in relation to breastfeeding and how these often work against and cause many barriers to breastfeeding. The breastfeeding support ingredients that many other countries utilize are missing in action or are underutilized here in America. I will discuss the few breastfeeding support ingredients we do have in America and discuss how they need to improve and expand to better support *all* breastfeeding mothers and babies.

While I am an advocate for breastfeeding mothers, I am in no way disparaging formula-feeding mothers! I am certainly pro-choice on this matter. I realize there are reasons for not breastfeeding, and I do not blame individual mothers for the infant-feeding choices that our systems and country often force them to make by refusing to adequately support breastfeeding mothers. I also want to add that breastfeeding is not a cure-all and doesn't solve all problems or illnesses, but it is a potent public health tool that is being grossly underutilized, undermeasured, undervalued, and undersupported.

Underlined words throughout this book will be defined in the glossary at the end of the book for easy reference. Also, I have placed all the referenced books, literature, and websites used in researching and writing this book at the end, organized by chapter and subject.

Support—The Key Ingredient Needed for Breastfeeding Success

America's expectation that mothers should breastfeed their babies—while it neglects to give them the support they need—results in mothers shouldering all the work of breastfeeding. Many moms experience regret and even guilt for not meeting their breastfeeding goals, but the blame lies with our country, institutions, and medical care system, which fail to support breastfeeding mothers and even create additional barriers. Currently, two-thirds of mothers in the US are not meeting their personal breastfeeding goals, and we as a nation are not meeting our national breastfeeding goals.

Breastfeeding goals are objectives for how long babies breastfeed (typically measured by whether the baby breastfeeds exclusively or partially, whether the baby breastfeeds within the first few hours after birth, and whether the baby has continued to breastfeed at three months, six months, and 12 months of age). Breastfeeding goals refer to personal goals that are measured by individuals and their doctors, and they also refer to national goals tracked by organizations like the Centers for Disease Control and Prevention (CDC) and Healthy People. Our national breastfeeding goals are not very high—I would say they are rather paltry—and our assessment of breastfeeding statistics related to our goals are unsatisfactory, as I will discuss later in this book. The Healthy People 2020 national breastfeeding goals are:

- Babies who breastfeed *at all*: 81.9%
- Babies who are still breastfeeding at *six months* of age: 60.6%
- Babies who are still breastfeeding at *one year* of age: 34.1%
- Babies who are *exclusively* breastfeeding at *three months* of age: 46.2%
- Babies who are *exclusively* breastfeeding at *six months* of age: 25.5%

Ideally, for the best health, babies should breastfeed exclusively in the first six months and continue breastfeeding for up to two years or more. This ensures the best health protections for both the baby and the mother.

Around two-thirds of mothers and babies do not breastfeed for as long as they intend or are recommended because they are not receiving the support they need and deserve. The top reasons mothers are not breastfeeding (or are not breastfeeding long enough to obtain significant benefits) are:

1. A lack of breastfeeding education, assessment, and documentation of breastfeeding status on every mother and baby.
2. A lack of accurate and comprehensive breastfeeding data and research to guide the management of this important public health issue.
3. A lack of timely and easily accessible breastfeeding support, services, and care providers (lactation consultants).
4. Overly medicalized childbirth interventions and too-frequent mother/infant separation in hospitals that do not adequately support breastfeeding.
5. A lack of pediatric-associated and community lactation services.
6. A lack of paid family leave, causing mothers to return to work too early before breastfeeding is well established.
7. The enticement and overuse of "free" commonly promoted formula from the medical care system and the Special Supplemental Nutrition Program for Women, Infants, and Children (WIC), and the social promotion of formula due to the USA's refusal to adopt the World Health Organization's (WHO) International Code of Marketing of Breast-milk Substitutes.

We also need to acknowledge that the many generations of not breastfeeding in our culture has had an <u>epigenetic</u> impact on some mothers' ability to breastfeed, increasing <u>metabolic diseases</u> and other <u>chronic illnesses</u> that cause breastfeeding problems. One baby not being breastfed doesn't result in the loss of the ability to breastfeed, but the mother who was not breastfed by the grandmother who was not breastfed by the great-grandmother who was not breastfed has a much higher risk of not being able to successfully breastfeed. This is due to the much higher <u>incidence</u> of metabolic disease and other diseases that result from generations of non-breastfeeding. Metabolic disease includes <u>obesity</u>, heart disease, high blood pressure, fertility problems, and diabetes, all of which cause breastfeeding problems. Just like the issue of weight gain and loss ("a minute on your lips, forever on your hips"), the issues caused by several generations of formula feeding and non-breastfeeding take a lot of work to undo, and it's going to take *lots of support* to get more babies back to the breast in America and keep them there for greater <u>dose-related benefits</u>! It will also take time, but if we don't start *now* to seriously expand and increase breastfeeding support in America, we are going to be further entrenched in the chronic illnesses that result from generations of non-breastfeeding. We already spend much more than any other country on medical care per person, yet do not enjoy the better health we deserve from that expenditure. Breastfeeding success following good support will help us turn that around.

Breastfeeding: A Key Ingredient for Health

We know how important having clean water and good nutrition is to our health and how these basics are responsible for most of our public health achievements. <u>Breast milk</u> is the best liquid nutrition for babies: filtered and enriched through the mother's body, made specially for them by their mother's attuned system, and adapted to suit their unique needs relative to their age and environment! It is also a lot more: it is a living and responsive immunizing medicine packaged in a rich <u>microbiome</u> that is <u>bioactive</u>, directive, adaptive, and dynamic, and is the foundation for good health, growth and development, and immune system function. It is an important system of nurturance, communication, sensory-rich stimulation, and an effective comforting/mothering tool between mamma and baby. It benefits mothers and others by saving time and resources and enhancing the satisfaction of the mom/baby relationship when it is going well. It is both a *multifactorial health tool and a health indicator* for both mother and baby!

Breastfeeding is a potent and vital health tool that needs and deserves recognition, protection, promotion, and support! I will discuss the identified problems/barriers to breastfeeding and make suggestions on how they can be reduced so that mothers and babies can enjoy more breastfeeding success and benefits. This book will elucidate how our country, systems, laws, policies, employers, health/medical care system, and communities can and should make it easier for mothers who want to breastfeed their babies so that the many moms who are not meeting their breastfeeding goals can be more successful with breastfeeding. I want to convince you of why and how breastfeeding should be a top national and medical priority with government and health care system recognition, resources, and funding to promote and support it. This "recipe for breastfeeding support" in America is for all who care about mothers and babies, so we can all enjoy the benefits of improved breastfeeding success rates with less regret and more confidence!

Breastfeeding is fundamental to the following:

1. Physiological Health
2. Developmental and Mental Health
3. Gender, Work, Racial, and Health Equity
4. Economic Health
5. Environmental Health
6. Maternal Empowerment
7. Social Health

This book contains seven chapters covering these categories of breastfeeding benefits and the major breastfeeding barriers, but it will not be an exhaustive coverage of all the issues. I will use what I have learned from my experience and work with breastfeeding mothers to illuminate major issues that need to be addressed. I will explain why and what we need to do to gain and maximize benefits from breastfeeding as a country. This book is a recipe for breastfeeding support in America from *all spheres of society*. Everyone benefits from breastfeeding success, as I will point out, and everyone needs to play an active role in breastfeeding support, giving relief to our breastfeeding mothers who are currently shouldering the important work of breastfeeding without the support they need and deserve. This book holds information for mothers, their supporters, health care providers and administrators, insurance companies, people serving in legislative capacity, lawyers, employers, and business and community leaders. I hope this book will be used as a recipe to improve our nation's health and well-being with these *ingredients of breastfeeding support,* which are central to a *key ingredient of health: breastfeeding.*

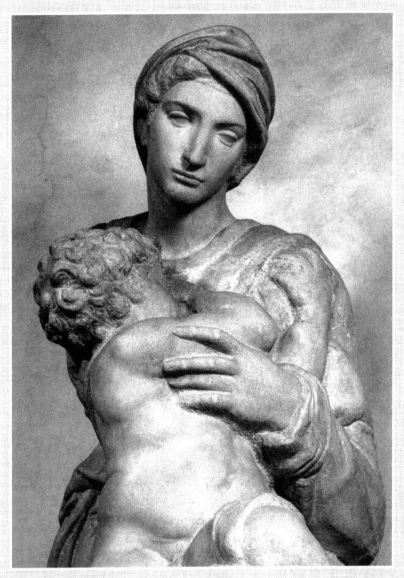

Turning to find the beloved breast: the *Medici Madonna* is a marble sculpture carved by Italian Renaissance master Michelangelo Buonarroti, demonstrating one of his favorite subjects, the nursing Virgin. Made in the early 16th century, this sculpture is now a piece of the altar decoration in the Basilica of St. Lawrence in Florence, Italy.

Physiological Health

Breastfeeding is a potent public health ingredient benefitting mothers' and babies' long-term health in many ways. It is what female bodies were designed to do after birth and what human babies need to be healthy and maximize their potential. When breastfeeding is not done, or is only done for a short time, it leads to an array of health-related problems. Our many years of being a formula/bottle-feeding country has been a huge factor in the many chronic health problems that we currently suffer from in America. Our exorbitant medical care costs in America are related to our low breastfeeding rates in the 20th century. Our focus on the products to feed our babies blinds us to the processes that breastfeeding entails. In this chapter, I will focus on an overview with a few chosen examples of the health conditions related to breastfeeding and how they are affected by not breastfeeding.

Breastfeeding protects and improves the <u>acute health</u>, or short-term health, of babies. While they are breastfeeding, babies get sick less frequently and less seriously from diarrheal, respiratory, viral and bacterial, ear, and other infections. When babies are less sick, and sick less often, it is a great relief to the parents and the whole family. That means a lot less suffering, less time out from daily life, and less medical bills, and it means babies can devote a lot more energy to growth and development. All babies get sick, but well-breastfed babies (generally meaning <u>fully breastfed</u> or mostly breastfed for around a year or more) get sick less often and less seriously. Breastfeeding's effects of reducing acute childhood illnesses and <u>infant mortality rates</u> are both well established and researched.

Breastfeeding benefits are dose-related, meaning the longer breastfeeding continues (and the more exclusively and intensively the baby is breastfed), the greater the protection both babies and mothers receive against chronic illnesses such as obesity, diabetes, heart disease, many cancers, and autoimmune illnesses. In American medicine, we do an adequate job managing short-term (acute) illnesses, but we are doing very poorly at managing chronic illnesses, which are much more disabling and costly than acute, short-term illnesses. Diabetes, heart disease, obesity, and hormonally related cancers are some of our top killers and cost the US the most in health care dollars, human suffering, and lost productivity. These illnesses are all a part of what is called metabolic syndrome/disease, which involves central (abdominal) obesity, insulin resistance, high blood pressure, abnormal cholesterol, and blood lipids. Metabolic syndrome and these accompanying diseases have significantly increased in the last century, coinciding with the rise of formula feeding, fast/junk food, and an inactive lifestyle in America. Formula is a baby's version of a highly processed junk food, and since it is given at the most vulnerable and fastest developmental stage of life, it has a greater negative health impact than junk food later on in a person's life.

How breastfeeding helps moms and babies avoid many chronic illnesses is under-researched, underappreciated, underreported, and under-taught in our medical/health system. For an example of how breastfeeding reduces chronic diseases, I will talk about its effect on the incidence of diabetes, obesity, and metabolic disease. Metabolic disease and diabetes cause multisystem illness and disability and are at epidemic proportions in the US. Diabetes is costing us more than one of every ten health care dollars in the US. It is one of our most expensive illnesses, with increasing incidence and rising costs projected (a projected incidence of up to 33% by 2050, according to the CDC). The WHO has also declared obesity as one of the most significant human health problems, with the expectation that 80% of women will be overweight (BMI of 25–29) or obese (BMI >30) by 2020! Obesity greatly increases the risk of diabetes and other metabolic diseases.

Breastfeeding reduces obesity and diabetes for both mom and baby by significant amounts if they are able to more fully breastfeed and continue breastfeeding for six months or more. Exclusive breastfeeding for the first six months of a baby's life, then continuing to breastfeed for another six months or more while adding foods, reduces the risk of the baby and mother developing obesity, diabetes, and the closely related metabolic disease by significant amounts—as much as 30% to 40% by some reports. Following is the explanation of how breastfeeding reduces diabetes, obesity, and metabolic disease risk and incidence both in a baby and a mother.

Breastfeeding: A Mom's Special Recipe

A breastfeeding baby grows and thrives on around 16% to 20% fewer calories than a formula-feeding baby because breast milk is customized, bioactive, dynamic, and much more bioavailable than formula, containing many hundreds of living ingredients. <u>Bioavailability</u> is the degree to which nutrients, probiotics, hormones, and neurochemicals are available for absorption and utilization in the body. Formula only has about 30 to 35 highly processed, hard to assimilate, nonliving ingredients and is the same recipe for every feed and every baby. Breast milk, though, is unique from each mother to each unique baby and adapts to the age and gender of the baby, the time of day, and different environments, including how the baby grows and develops and whether the baby is healthy or has an illness. Even the way a baby breastfeeds helps to determine the specific "recipe" of the mother's milk!

As Maureen Minchin, the author of *Milk Matters*, says, "A mother's own milk, fed from her own body, has been the physiological norm since mammals evolved millions of years ago. The milk of each species has evolved to perfectly suit that species … and individual mothers of that species produce milk tailored both for that child and for the environment in which they and their infant live."

Katie Hinde, an anthropologist, in her TED talk about mother's milk, discusses the biological recipe for breast milk as variable and different by age and development of baby, time of day, location where mom and baby live, and even for girl babies and boy babies because girls and boys have different growth rates and patterns! Formula is a one-type-fits-all, nonliving recipe with few ingredients, while breast milk is a mom's unique recipe for her unique baby! Breastfeeding is also much more than just good nutrition and immunity protection—as Katie Hinde states in her TED talk, "Milk doesn't just grow the body; it fuels behavior and shapes neurodevelopment."

E. A. Quinn, an anthropologist at Washington University in St. Louis, MO, has done research on the variability of a mother's milk in different environments and at different altitudes. Her research has even shown how the breastfeeding mother's length of being breastfed herself has an effect on her lactation experience!

Breast milk's unique recipe means that because a mom's milk is so much more bioavailable to the baby, it is a *"less is more"* form of nourishment. The breastfed baby, having a reduced caloric intake (yet full of bioactive nutrients) compared to formula-fed babies, grows and develops much better on fewer calories. This is a significant factor in protection from obesity and diabetes for babies. Also, breastfeeding babies work for their food, so they are not as likely to overfeed, but with bottle feeding, overfeeding is common. Another reason babies who are formula fed have greater risk of obesity and diabetes later in life might be because a first and/or foremost ingredient of many formulas is corn syrup. (I will give a list of typical formula ingredients later in this book.) Another reason formula increases the risk of diabetes is that it might cause an immune system reaction due to foreign proteins based on cow's milk proteins, which are meant to grow a very different (and larger) animal.

We know that metabolic and nutritional habits begin in infancy, so that means breastfed babies are at a lower risk for poor eating habits that can result in obesity (and all the other chronic illnesses that accompany obesity, including diabetes). The improved intestinal flora (gut microbiome) and immune function of the breastfed baby, due to the alive prebiotics and probiotics, and the dynamic aspects of breast milk also contribute to the reduction of the risk of obesity and diabetes.

The Metabolic Stimulation of Breastfeeding for the Mother

For the mother, because breastfeeding acts as a daily metabolic stimulant, it reduces her risk of obesity/metabolic disease and their tagalong, diabetes—and the risk reduction adds up with each month and each baby she breastfeeds. *Breastfeeding is a potent form of metabolic stimulation, just like exercise*! Breastfeeding mothers burn an average of a quarter of a million calories in one year of <u>fully breastfeeding</u>. This daily and sustained metabolic stimulation is a significant, but underappreciated and under-researched, factor in reducing a mother's risk of obesity and diabetes. The approximately 250,000 calories burned in a year of breastfeeding are roughly equivalent to running 400 to 450 miles or walking 1,000 miles. This milk making/calorie burning is a significant daily metabolic boost that decreases a mother's risk of many other chronic illnesses as well, like hypertension and heart disease. Breastfeeding is a wonderful opportunity for a woman to significantly boost her metabolic rate for a *sustained time*, which is so important in our metabolically understimulating modern lifestyle!

A mother who breastfeeds not only increases her metabolism by burning calories to make milk, she also increases her physical movement and muscle work through breastfeeding. The physical act of breastfeeding is a form of bodily exercise for the mother that helps reestablish a more physically active lifestyle incorporating movement and production instead of outsourcing it. Think of the thousands of times a mother picks up her baby, positions, holds, and carries the baby to breastfeed over a year, or more, of time. All mothers pick up and carry their babies, but breastfeeding mothers do so much more often as it is necessary for the act of direct breastfeeding. The baby who breastfeeds is also more physically active through the many changing positions, greater interactivity with mother, and the greater oral and physical work of breastfeeding. All this calorie burning and bodily movement add up over the many days and months of breastfeeding and help offset the diseases of inactivity so prevalent in these modern times.

If a mother breastfeeds more than one baby, the protections and benefits are cumulative. Recent research demonstrates that mothers with gestational diabetes (diabetes during pregnancy) who breastfeed for at least six months can have a 47% reduced risk of diabetes later in life due to the sustained metabolic stimulation of breastfeeding. Imagine the reduction of diabetes risk if she breastfeeds three babies for a year each!

Diabetes and obesity are just two examples of how breastfeeding reduces the incidence of chronic disease. Breastfeeding also reduces the incidence and/or severity of many other illnesses, such as cancers, cardiovascular diseases, autoimmune diseases, infectious diseases, developmental problems, and gastrointestinal diseases. If I were to cover all these diseases, this book would be very long, so I am just focusing on diabetes, metabolic syndrome, and obesity here as examples of how important breastfeeding is for a mother's and baby's long-term health!

It is important to note that breastfeeding benefits are *dose-related*: the more exclusively and longer the breastfeeding continues, the more benefits the mother and baby will both gain for the rest of their lives. A few days or weeks of breastfeeding (<u>token breastfeeding</u>) is not going to garner dose-related long-term benefits. Sadly, because almost two-thirds of mothers and babies <u>wean</u> earlier than they intend and are recommended to, many are not able to maximize these long-term protections against chronic illnesses. It would help to know more about and exactly when and why mothers wean from breastfeeding so we could direct our efforts to address those issues. Unfortunately, we do not have comprehensive breastfeeding data in the US because we don't have a system for assessing and recording data on all breastfeeding mothers and babies.

The Breastfeeding Data and the Breastfeeding Report Card

The management of any issue begins with accurate, comprehensive, and timely assessment. The data obtained from assessment then leads to the solutions for and management of that issue. There is a serious lack of timely breastfeeding data on mothers and babies in our health/medical care system. This is one area of health care data that has been unwisely ignored.

The World Health Organization recommends breastfeeding for two years, but in the US, we wean our babies from the breast much sooner, with around 84% women initiating breastfeeding but barely 36% still breastfeeding at one year, which is the end point of any breastfeeding assessment in the US. These low breastfeeding continuation rates are indicative that America is making it too hard for mothers to breastfeed for the recommended longer periods of time. These statistics come from the CDC's Breastfeeding Report Card. Yet these breastfeeding statistics are really only an estimate, and we don't know much about exactly when and why mothers wean their babies from the breast sooner than the recommended goal and incidence of one to two years.

Even though breastfeeding is known to be a potent public health tool, we don't comprehensively or accurately assess and document breastfeeding rates in the US! The Breastfeeding Report Card data come from a small retrospective phone survey for immunization statistics *(less than 1% of the population is surveyed, and this phone survey occurs 19 to 35 months after the baby's birth)*. These surveys are not even dedicated to breastfeeding assessment and only have four breastfeeding-related questions tacked on at the end after many questions about man-made/medical immunizations.

How can we know if we are improving our rates of breastfeeding (as recommended by our national health goals) if we do not have a comprehensive and accurate method of assessing and amassing timely breastfeeding statistics?

How do we count the work of breastfeeding and plan for breastfeeding support if breastfeeding is not even accurately counted?

How do we manage and plan for the need for breastfeeding support if we don't even accurately, timely, and comprehensively measure breastfeeding statuses on all babies?

Estimates based on a small and late phone survey are not an adequate assessment for the important public health tool of breastfeeding. We need to treat breastfeeding as a vital sign and key health indicator just like weight, length, temperature, blood pressure, and other health measurements! Breastfeeding assessment documentation needs to be made data-friendly so it can be collected and used. We do a good job of man-made immunizations, collecting the data (for local, state, national, and educational agencies) and documenting every medical immunization on a baby's individual health care records and for school records. Breastfeeding provides the first and foremost immunization of a baby as the immunities pass from the mother's mature immune system through her milk to her baby's immature system. It makes sense that we should assess and document breastfeeding (mom-made) immunization data on the medical record at every well-baby visit at the same time we give and document medical (man-made) immunization data. Four questions asked and the answers documented at every well-baby medical visit would give us accurate breastfeeding initiation, exclusivity or partiality, and duration data:

1. How many times does the baby breastfeed directly in 24 hours?
2. How many ounces of expressed, pumped, banked, or donor breast milk is the baby receiving in 24 hours?
3. How many ounces of formula or other liquids is the baby receiving in 24 hours?
4. When were foods introduced, and how many times in 24 hours is the baby fed solid foods?

These four questions should be asked by the health care provider or staff at every well-baby visit for at least the first two years, and the answers should be recorded on the baby's chart. This would give specific information about how much and how long the baby is breastfed (including exclusive, partial, short-term, or extended breastfeeding) and if they are receiving formula to supplement, as well as how much formula, when formula was started, and when solid foods were started. Then this information can be collected and sent to the appropriate local, state, and federal agencies (like the CDC) along with the other immunization records, following HIPAA rules. That way, we would have *accurate, comprehensive, and real-time breastfeeding statistics* and could really see the effectiveness of breastfeeding as a public health tool, as well as where exactly we need to devote our resources to enhance breastfeeding support efforts. Adding these four questions to the baby's electronic health record (EHR) and to the mother's chart when she is seen by her health care provider would give accurate, comprehensive, timely breastfeeding data. Breastfeeding data is important for both the mother and the baby and for our health care system! Breastfeeding is an important but overlooked vital sign and key health indicator that deserves comprehensive and accurate assessment and documentation! It is a potent health care tool for both mother and baby, and it deserves to be accurately counted so it can be better managed! Mothers also deserve to have their work of breastfeeding recognized and documented, and hopefully it will lead to paid family leave and other needed breastfeeding resources.

Asking these questions would also help to identify the mothers needing a referral to a <u>lactation professional</u>, thereby helping to reduce the earlier-than-intended breastfeeding cessation that often happens due to untreated breastfeeding problems. The questions that get asked get more attention and recognition in our health care system! It has been wisely stated, "*You don't count until you are counted,*" or in this case, "*Your breastfeeding doesn't count until it is counted.*" What is not assessed, counted, and documented cannot be managed within our health care system and society.

Evidence-based breastfeeding data correlated with outcomes would lead to greater investment and expansion of breastfeeding support at *all* levels of society: trained health and lactation care providers, breastfeeding-friendly hospitals; breastfeeding-friendly employers and day care providers, businesses, and products; breastfeeding-friendly pediatric, postpartum, and family planning care; nursing in public protective national laws and policies; insurance coverage for breastfeeding services; breastfeeding-friendly support in communities; and national paid family leave (discussed in Chapter 3).

The following is based on a poster presentation I gave at the 2017 Breastfeeding and Feminism International Conference regarding this issue of breastfeeding statistics. The Breastfeeding and Feminism International Conference is held every year in the Raleigh-Durham-Chapel Hill metropolitan region in North Carolina and is one of the few conferences that address the issues of breastfeeding support, laws, policies, funding, research, and cultural and systemic differences in breastfeeding practices around the world.

What Is Measured Matters and What Matters Should Be Measured

Breastfeeding is unique to a woman and, as many women's issues, has been relegated to the unrecognized "women's work" by our health care system and society. However, breastfeeding is an important indicator and promoter of health status, and it needs accurate and comprehensive assessment, documentation, and monitoring. Action 19 of the 2011 Surgeon General's "Call to Action to Support Breastfeeding" called for the development of a national monitoring system to improve the tracking of breastfeeding rates as well as the policies and environmental factors that affect breastfeeding. Breastfeeding data in the Unites States is currently collected in different ways. My presentation described the various ways we collect breastfeeding data and the weaknesses and strengths of these various methods. It concluded with specific recommendations for an improved manner of collecting and documenting breastfeeding status of all babies in the US.

Critique of Current Breastfeeding Report Card Statistics Assessment Methods

Data from two sources, the National Immunization Survey (NIS) and Maternity Practices in Infant Nutrition and Care (mPINC), are used by the Centers for Disease Control and Prevention to create the Breastfeeding Report Card every two years. There are some other breastfeeding assessment tools but nothing that is specific to breastfeeding, and they are all different, with different questions, and their results are conflicting and so are not used in the Breastfeeding Report Card. The history of breastfeeding assessment came from Ross formula labs to assess the competition (breastfeeding) for their product—imagine letting a formula company be the only source of breastfeeding statistics until 2001! WIC also assesses breastfeeding status and covers over 50% of mothers and babies in America; however, the WIC breastfeeding assessment is attached to a benefit/food package and is easily manipulated to get a certain kind of food package, which also leads to inaccurate breastfeeding statistics. Below is the critique of the two sources of breastfeeding data that are used for the **CDC's Breastfeeding Report Card:**

Assessment Tool	Strengths	Weaknesses
National Immunization Survey (NIS)	Started in 2001, performed by CDC every two years, phone survey of parents of 19- to 35-month-old babies, population-based with random sampling.	Small phone survey of <1% of population, retrospective 19–35 months after birth, not specific to breastfeeding, and too meager—only four breastfeeding questions at the end of a large immunization survey, changed over the years, causing interpretation problems.
Maternity Practices in Infant Nutrition and Care (mPINC)	Started in 2007, performed by CDC every two years in all hospitals in the US that do labor and delivery care. Good survey of breastfeeding support in postpartum/hospital setting and assesses data on initiation of breastfeeding practices.	Does not assess or include any breastfeeding continuation statistics or breastfeeding practices and support outside of hospital setting.

To summarize: These breastfeeding assessment tools do not address the need for real-time, ongoing, accurate, comprehensive, and continuing breastfeeding statistics that are needed to document and monitor the breastfeeding status of all American mothers and babies!

Real-Time, Accurate, and Comprehensive Breastfeeding Statistics

Since breastfeeding is a "mom-made" immunization, and since man-made immunizations are assessed in a systemic and accurate manner at all well-baby visits, I recommend that breastfeeding statistics also be assessed at *all* well-baby visits via four questions:

1. How many times does the baby breastfeed directly in 24 hours?
2. How many ounces of expressed, pumped, banked, or donor breast milk is the baby receiving in 24 hours?
3. How many ounces of formula or other liquids is the baby receiving in 24 hours?
4. When were foods introduced, and how many times in 24 hours is the baby fed solid foods?

These questions would give exclusive, partial, and continued breastfeeding statistics on every baby in the well-baby care system and could easily be compiled by states and the CDC for accurate and comprehensive breastfeeding statistics to be used for comprehensive research related to breastfeeding benefits, used to move from assessment to referral for needed breastfeeding services, and used to support the reasons for more lactation professionals and paid family leave in America. It all starts with an accurate and comprehensive assessment and documentation of breastfeeding statistics!

How these real-time, comprehensive, and accurate breastfeeding data could be used:

Policy
- To accurately and comprehensively measure progress toward the national and state breastfeeding rates.
- To plan and review programs/policies aimed at increasing breastfeeding rates and duration.
- To increase breastfeeding support resources where needed.
- To document the need for more lactation professionals and funding to support their training.
- To guide insurance companies in recognizing the need for reimbursement for lactation services.
- To document the work mothers are doing to breastfeed their babies.
- To support the need and reasons for, and expected cost savings for, paid family leave in the US.

Clinical
- To identify breastfeeding problems earlier and facilitate early referrals to a lactation professional if needed before an earlier-than-intended weaning occurs.
- To increase attention to the importance and clinical significance of breastfeeding—the question that gets asked gets attention by both client and health care provider!

Research
- To investigate breastfeeding as it relates to health and illness issues in maternal/infant health.
- To facilitate breastfeeding research with the use of breastfeeding data.

The Baby-Friendly Hospital Initiative (BFHI)

In 1991, WHO and UNICEF began the Baby-Friendly Hospital Initiative (BFHI) as a global response to medical policies and practices that had negative effects on breastfeeding initiation during birth and postpartum hospital stays. The BFHI addresses the problems of there being too few lactation professionals to support the breastfeeding mom and baby in the hospital; doctors, nurses, and other hospital staff who lack breastfeeding education and practice in such a manner that thwarts mothers' efforts to breastfeed; separation of moms and babies, which causes babies not to breastfeed often enough; medicines that reduce breast milk production; medical interventions that have a negative effect on breastfeeding; and the use of free formula in hospitals. However, today, there are way too few Baby-Friendly hospitals in the US.

The Baby-Friendly Hospital Initiative encourages hospitals to help mothers breastfeed by meeting 10 standards:

1. Have a written breastfeeding policy.
2. Train all involved health care providers.
3. Inform all mothers about breastfeeding.
4. Help mothers get started with breastfeeding.
5. Teach mothers how to breastfeed effectively.
6. Give no formula unless medically prescribed or at mother's choice.
7. Provide 24-hour rooming-in.
8. Encourage breastfeeding on demand.
9. Give no artificial nipples.
10. Refer mothers to timely and accessible breastfeeding support in the community.

The BFHI also mandates that certified birthing facilities follow the World Health Organization's International Code of Marketing of Breast-milk Substitutes, which mandates hospitals to pay fully for the formula they use instead of getting free formula from the formula companies as they always have in the past.

The BFHI is only actively in effect in 539 hospitals in the United States, representing only 26.8% of all births in the US, even though it clearly needs to be in every hospital that serves mothers and babies. It also needs to expand its reach to include addressing the following:

1. Overuse of intravenous fluids during labor and delivery
2. Overuse of Pitocin during labor and delivery and postpartum
3. Circumcisions being performed on newborn boys who have not gotten breastfeeding well established on second day of life, not giving them enough time to recover from birth
4. Undiagnosed and untreated tongue-ties leading to breastfeeding problems and early weaning after discharge
5. Overuse of medical procedures (including epidurals and C-sections) that could be avoided by better obstetrical management and active support of the mother during her labor from doulas, lactation professionals, and other helpful staff

Overuse of intravenous (IV) fluids during birth causes mothers to experience more breast engorgement, leading to difficulties with latching and damaged, sore nipples, which is a big reason why women stop breastfeeding in the early weeks. The reason laboring women need so much IV fluids is because of the early and common use of epidurals in most births. Overuse of IV fluids also overhydrates babies and causes babies' postbirth (fluid) weight loss to seem greater when babies diurese after birth through urination. This perceived weight loss, of course, leads to greater formula supplementation. New lactation policies suggest making the baby's weight at 24 hours post birth the baseline weight for determining weight gain to compensate for the problem of overhydration. Only a few hospitals have enacted this policy, though.

The BFHI also needs to expand their policies to address the overuse of Pitocin, the artificial/man-made version of oxytocin, to induce/augment labor and for postpartum uterine contractility. Pitocin is commonly used in American birth practices to compensate for the slowing of labor due to epidural usage. Pitocin is also often given before due dates when a woman's body is not ripe for labor! Its use necessitates extra and earlier usage of epidurals and more IV fluids and strict bedrest for laboring women—being in bed is the worst place for a woman in labor! It is overused, and its ill effects are under-elucidated. It is important to remember that when Pitocin is used to hurry up a labor, even though an epidural is used to relieve the pain, the woman's and baby's bodies are suffering from the harder work of an induced labor! Consequently, the mom and baby who were induced are often physically exhausted and need more medical interventions to treat the more common fevers and higher blood pressures in the postpartum course after inductions. Pitocin is also administered immediately post-birth to contract the uterus, but putting the baby immediately to breastfeed contracts the uterus naturally, so Pitocin is not needed unless the mother chooses not to breastfeed.

Another ill effect of Pitocin is that it often causes mothers to have delayed milk production, leading to greater needs for babies to be supplemented. Pitocin is also an antidiuretic, adding to the problem of edema and engorgement of the breasts caused by overuse of IV fluids coupled with the antidiuretic effect. The heavy and common use of Pitocin negatively affects breastfeeding initiation for many reasons, and the BFHI needs to address this!

And, most importantly and urgently, the BFHI needs to address the issue of baby boys being circumcised, as <u>circumcision</u> has a negative effect on a baby's breastfeeding frequency and effectiveness. Circumcision surgery removes the foreskin that covers and protects the tip of the penis. It is usually done on the second day of life before a newborn leaves the hospital. Most babies in the world are not circumcised, and most experts around the world feel that hygiene is sufficient and circumcision is not a medical necessity. As with all surgical procedures, there are risks, and the surgery is painful during and after the procedure until it heals. It often interferes with breastfeeding by causing the baby to miss breastfeeds due to being away from the mother for the procedure and being too upset to feed well for a while after the procedure.

When I worked in a hospital as a lactation consultant, I noticed that baby boys who had been circumcised often did not breastfeed for six to eight hours after the circumcision! This delay in breastfeeding frequency on the second day of life (when most circumcisions are done) delays a mother's milk production, causes greater infant weight loss, and increases use of formula supplementation, thereby decreasing a mother's chances for breastfeeding success. I feel if parents want their baby boy to be circumcised (which is not a medical necessity), they should do it after breastfeeding is well established as an outpatient procedure. Babies experience enough challenges and pain from birth, and they should not have to endure the pain of unnecessary, barbaric medical procedures in addition!

On another subject regarding medical procedures that might be needed after a baby is born and before the baby is discharged are the underrecognized and undertreated tongue-ties, which affect around 10% of newborns, with boys being affected more often. A tongue-tie means that the frenulum is too restrictive and the tongue cannot move in order to effectively breastfeed. Mothers who try to breastfeed a baby with a tongue-tie most often get sore and traumatized nipples, which is a serious deterrent to breastfeeding. A frenectomy (clipping of the frenulum) is often medically necessary and a much easier and less-invasive procedure than a circumcision, yet frenectomies are done less often. Many babies are discharged with an untreated, tight frenulum, making breastfeeding impossible or very painful for the mother. These tongue-ties need to be treated before the newborn is discharged, yet most doctors are unfamiliar with how to do this simple procedure.

More complicated frenectomies (such as for posterior tongue-ties, which require laser treatment) may require treatment after the baby has been discharged from the hospital, but simple anterior frenectomies should be treated at the hospital before discharge so these babies can successfully breastfeed. All obstetric (OB) and pediatric doctors need to be taught in their medical education programs how to do frenectomies! Not doing the necessary frenectomies before discharge dooms the mother to breastfeeding difficulties and pain, the newborn to greater weight loss and higher risk of jaundice, and both to the greater risk of breastfeeding failure and all the risks of greater illness that come with that.

We need to recognize that a medicalized birth with use of IV fluids, medicines, and procedures such as epidurals, vacuum-assisted deliveries, C-sections, and circumcisions help medical care providers and hospital systems make more money, offsetting the fact that normal OB services are generally a money loser for the hospitals. Our for-profit medical system in the US lends itself to the encouragement of a medicalized birth rather than devoting more providers and resources to promoting more natural births. Natural births, with more hands-on care such as doulas give, are better for getting breastfeeding off to an easier start, while medicalized births often lead to the medicalized form of infant feeding: formula feeding. And formula feeding leads to the need for more medical care due to causing more illness for mothers and babies, resulting in more tertiary-care profits. It's all related, and the Baby-Friendly Hospital Initiative (BFHI) really needs to expand its reach and focus to address these issues (IV fluid and Pitocin overuse, medicalized births, and circumcisions), which are barriers to breastfeeding!

The WHO Code

The WHO Code (or "the Code") was adopted in 1981 by the World Health Assembly (WHA) to promote safe and beneficial nutrition for infants by the protection and promotion of breastfeeding and by ensuring the proper use of breast milk substitutes if they are medically necessary. Because of the vulnerability of infants and the health risks due to unnecessary or improper use of breast milk substitutes, the marketing of formula and breast milk substitutes requires special restrictions. Casual and common marketing practices are unsuitable for formulas and breast milk substitutes. This issue of restrictions for formula marketing is similar to the restriction of tobacco advertising in the US due to the fact that cigarette smoking/tobacco is so toxic and causes so much illness, death, and higher medical costs. Formula use, especially in areas of the world where there is a lack of clean water and refrigeration, results in much higher rates of infant mortality!

This WHO Code restricting the marketing practices of formula has been adopted by around 136 of the 194 WHO member countries. Most have enacted legislation implementing many, or at least some, of the provisions of the Code. Only 46 member states have nonlegal or no measures in place, and the US is one of them.

The main restrictions required in the Code include:

- no advertising of breast milk substitutes and other related products to the public;
- no free samples to mothers, their families, or health care workers; no free or discounted formula;
- no promotion of products: no product displays or distribution of promotional materials;
- no donations of free or subsidized supplies of breast milk substitutes or related products in any part of the health care system;
- no company-paid personnel to contact or to advise mothers or health care workers;
- no gifts or personal samples to health care workers;
- no pictures or text idealizing artificial feeding on the labels of the products;
- information to health workers should only be scientific and factual;
- information on artificial feeding should explain the importance of breastfeeding, and the health hazards and increased costs associated with artificial feeding;
- all products should be of a high quality, and unsuitable products, such as sweetened condensed milk, should not be allowed.

The US has taken *never* taken *any* action on the Code in this country (as easily evidenced by the ads on TV and in newspapers and grocery store ads for formulas). It is also common that formula companies get a newly pregnant woman's information through gift registries at stores and from doctors' offices. Then they start receiving free coupons and ads for formula during their pregnancy.

At the most recent 2018 World Health Assembly meeting, US Health and Human Services (HHS) tried to use its influence to decrease protections that the Code embodied for breastfeeding protection in *other* countries in the interest of promoting "choice" for mothers in those countries. The following is from an article in *The Atlantic* called "The Epic Battle Between Breast Milk and Infant-Formula Companies" by Olga Khazan, dated Jul 10, 2018:

> The American delegates wanted to ditch language in the nonbinding resolution that called on governments to "protect, promote, and support breastfeeding" and another passage that called on policymakers to restrict the promotion of unhealthy food products. When that didn't work, they threatened Ecuador, the country that intended to introduce the breastfeeding measure, with punitive trade and aid measures. Ultimately, it was Russia that agreed to introduce the breastfeeding resolution, and the U.S.'s efforts were "largely unsuccessful," the *Times* reported.

Caitlyn Oakley, HHS national spokesperson, denied that the US did this, stating, "The United States was fighting to protect women's abilities to make the best choices for the nutrition of their babies," but there were many speakers at the WHA who spoke out against the action that the US took.

The representatives from Save the Children, World Cancer Research Fund International, International Union Against TB and Lung Disease, and other organizations who were in attendance at the WHA meeting expressed dismay at the weakening of the protections against the promotion of formula in the revised resolution. Following are three of the statements indicating this concern, taken from the document of the meetings about this "conflict of interest" resolution:

"The representative of the WORLD CANCER RESEARCH FUND INTERNATIONAL, speaking at the invitation of the CHAIRMAN, drew attention to his association's latest report on the links between cancer and diet, nutrition and physical activity. He expressed concern that the text of the revised draft resolution had been weakened. The fact that the drafting group had been unable to reaffirm commitment to implementing existing WHO guidance and policies was alarming. Member States should scale up effective interventions to prevent conflicts of interest in the policy development process with a view to increasing breastfeeding rates."

"The representative of the INTERNATIONAL UNION AGAINST TUBERCULOSIS AND LUNG DISEASE, speaking at the invitation of the CHAIRMAN, said that civil society no longer wished to see profits and commercial interests placed above the health of the vulnerable. Policies must protect children from conflicts of interest and industry interference. Low-cost interventions such as breastfeeding support were a wise investment in health. She supported the initial draft resolution, which had underscored the importance of protecting breastfeeding through legal measures and strengthened implementation of the Code. Like other recent attempts to regulate in that area, the revised draft resolution had been weakened to the point that it potentially compromised the health of millions of children."

"The representative of THE SAVE THE CHILDREN FUND, speaking at the invitation of the CHAIRMAN, urged States to invest further in nutrition to achieve Sustainable Development Goal 2 (End hunger, achieve food security and improved nutrition and promote sustainable agriculture). Costed and scaled-up nutrition plans should be financed and integrated into national strategies for universal health coverage. She urged Governments to prioritize breastfeeding, which they had a duty to protect, promote and support under the Convention on the Rights of the Child, and expressed concern that the marketing activities of some manufacturers and distributors put children at risk. While the Member States that had sponsored the original draft resolution should be commended, she expressed dismay at the weakening of the revised draft resolution and the inability of the drafting group to reaffirm commitments to implement existing WHO guidance and policies."

This lessening of the protections against advertising formula for young infants in the interest of "choice" is especially egregious when considering that, in many countries, there is inadequate access to clean water, refrigeration, medical care, and money to purchase the formula after they have lost their own milk supply. A formula-fed infant in these situations is much more likely to die than a breastfed infant! Why is the US trying to influence this policy elsewhere in the world, in addition to refusing to abide by it in our own country? The reason is that the US is supporting the formula industry's profits over the health and well-being of babies so that formula can be more easily sold and profited from in other countries. This is shameful!

Summary

In this first chapter, I've discussed just some of the physiological benefits of breastfeeding and the significant impact on reduction of the risk of metabolic disease, obesity, and diabetes for both mother and baby as one major example of the importance of breastfeeding. My recommendations for breastfeeding support "ingredients" include doing accurate and comprehensive breastfeeding assessment, documentation, and data collection on all babies; improving and making all birthing hospitals/centers "Baby Friendly"; reducing medicalization of births and infant care by enhancing childbirth and breastfeeding support in our hospitals; and enacting legislation and policy protecting against inappropriate marketing and promotion of formula using "the Code." These are some of the needed ingredients of breastfeeding support in America. More will be discussed in the following chapters.

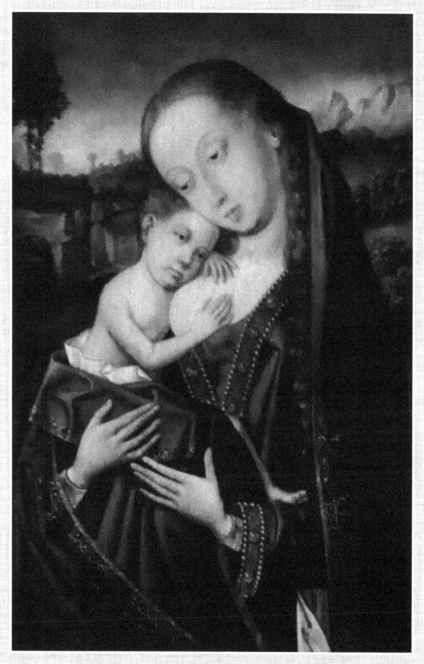

This painting by the artist known as the Master of the Legend of the Magdalen (1480–1537) depicts the love bond so well! The way to the baby's heart is through their stomach!

— 2 —

Developmental and Mental Health

Breastfeeding is an interactive delivery system. It requires frequent and close contact and thus is physically and emotionally interactive. <u>Direct breastfeeding</u> is an "in-your-face" activity that necessitates a physical closeness that lends itself to a relational closeness. In my work with mothers and babies, I see that breastfeeding mothers often smile and touch or talk to their babies while they are breastfeeding them, and babies often smile or reach up and touch their mother's face. This means that breastfed babies receive more interrelational, verbal, aural, visual, tactile, and kinesthetic stimulation early on, when their brains are developing at the fastest rate. Formula-feeding mothers and babies are less closely connected physically, and this means they are at risk of having less interactivity. Formula-feeding parents can approximate the interactivity of breastfeeding by holding their bottle-feeding baby close and interacting with them during the feeds, but it is tempting to do what I see some bottle-feeding caregivers do (no matter what is in the bottle), and that is to prop or let the baby hold the bottle, be less interactive with the baby during the feed, or let others feed the baby too often. Unfortunately, many mothers who have to return to work feel compelled to get their babies used to bottles so they can be fed by someone else when the mother is gone.

Directly breastfeeding mothers and babies can't prop the bottle, which is one reason direct breastfeeding is more beneficial than expressed/pumped breast milk feeding. Direct breastfeeding has a huge impact on the benefits derived from breastfeeding—because of greater communication between the mother's and baby's body and more interactivity. There is research on how a mother's milk recipe changes to meet her baby's needs, and direct breastfeeding is important for the communication between mother and baby to occur so the milk recipe can adapt to the baby's needs. Bottle-feeding pumped milk cuts out this important communication between mother and baby. Also, one of the most wonderful benefits of breastfeeding, *convenience*, is negated for the mother who has to spend time pumping milk, transferring it to bags for refrigeration or freezing, and then getting it out to warm and rebottle it, bottle-feed it to the baby, and clean pump parts and bottle after. The milk she pumped previously is most likely out of sync with the time of day and developmental or health state of her baby when the baby receives it. The better benefits from *direct* breastfeeding is another reason mothers need paid family leave to stay at home longer and not have to resort to pumped breast milk bottle-feeding or formula bottle-feeding, as it is not just what goes into the bottle but also the bottle-feeding itself that has fewer benefits.

Breastfeeding's specificity and made-to-demand/need type of nutrition is involved in better infant development, which is diminished when previously pumped milk is bottle-fed versus direct breastfeeding. Breastfeeding is dynamic and has a circadian rhythm to it, and its recipe changes according to the time of day and age and characteristics of the baby. Breast milk is alive and active, with hundreds of identified elements that aid digestion, facilitate absorption of nutrients, and serve to protect the baby's health. Recently, breast milk has been found to contain stem cells, which migrate from the gut to the brain, and this could be, in part, why breastfed children often do better in school. They also do better in school because they are sick less often and less seriously, allowing them to spend more time learning and developing.

Neuroprotective Effects

It has also been said that breastfeeding may reduce occurrence or delay onset of some of the mental and neurodevelopmental illnesses. Perhaps this is due to the better sensory stimulation, more bioavailable nutrients in breast milk, and facilitated bonding between mother and baby due to the connectivity of direct breastfeeding. For example, autism is now being diagnosed in as many as one in 68 children in the US. There is a large gastrointestinal component to this neurodevelopmental condition, and breastfeeding, with its living cells, immunity-building, and dynamic changes, helps to offset some of the potential problems associated with autism, and that, in turn, helps to decrease the needs for medical, educational, and social care services.

The biomechanical/physiological act of breastfeeding also comprises many "first-line" treatments for neurodevelopmental or behavioral issues, such as with prematurity, autism, or Down syndrome. This is because the sensory/relational stimulation and optimal nutrition and immune protection that afflicted babies receive from the onset of life sets the stage for the best outcome. Direct breastfeeding is nutritional therapy, physical therapy, occupational therapy, relational therapy, and speech therapy all in one! These are the therapies that are utilized for neurodevelopmental deficits, and with breastfeeding, they begin at birth. So, breastfed premature or developmentally challenged babies are getting the earliest treatment/therapy for developmental problems at their mother's breast.

Many neurodevelopmental or behavioral disorders are not discovered until later in life; yet with breastfeeding, babies are being treated early, even before diagnosis! Neurodevelopmental problems begin early in life and result in worse performance in school, less productive learning time, and possibly greater chances of getting kicked out of classes or even out of school due to behavioral problems associated with neurodevelopmental problems. If we collected enough comprehensive breastfeeding data, I wonder if we would see that formula-fed babies are more likely to have educational problems, especially when they suffer from poverty, medical, developmental, and social stresses. This is not to imply that all breastfed babies do well in school and all formula-fed babies grow up with problems. Rather, what I am saying is that the same kinds of barriers that result in low breastfeeding incidence also increase the risk of developmental and behavioral problems. Furthermore, the mothers and babies most at risk for these issues are the least likely to receive the support and services they need and deserve to succeed at breastfeeding to alleviate these same problems. They also receive less breastfeeding support due to so much time, energy, and funding being devoured by medical treatments resulting in the exclusion of breastfeeding support, even though breastfeeding support and success would rival as an effective treatment. Early and more intensive breastfeeding support and success help to ameliorate and give the most effective primary care for these problems through its many neurodevelopmental and psychosocial benefits, as described.

Early treatment of a deficit or problem is much less costly than tertiary medical care, and breastfeeding naturally encompasses this early and *primary* treatment, leading to better outcomes. However, babies with prematurity and/or neurodevelopmental disorders are often harder to breastfeed because of their issues, and their mothers need more support, assistance, and time with breastfeeding to help them be successful and reap the benefits of breastfeeding. This adds to our need for more lactation professionals and paid family leave in the US.

Successful breastfeeding is also said to reduce the incidence of postpartum depression (PPD) for mothers. We know that PPD is becoming more prevalent and is not good for the mother or baby because of less positive interaction from a depressed mother. Those mothers who suffer with PPD endure a stressful and unpleasant start on their mothering journey instead of enjoying and feeling empowered by it. Breastfeeding problems can increase the likelihood of PPD, but successful breastfeeding reduces PPD. The hormones of breastfeeding, prolactin and oxytocin, have positive behavioral effects for the breastfeeding mother, helping her to feel calmer and more tolerant of the stresses of new motherhood! These same hormones are in her milk as well and influence her baby's behavior to some degree also! There has been some study regarding how a mother's milk changes in relation to time of day and has more prolactin in it and melatonin at nighttime, helping her and her baby to sleep better. Sleep is, of course, very important to mental health and well-being! This is another reason to give more breastfeeding support: so mothers can be successful with breastfeeding and gain the benefit of improved mental health as they begin this important job of mothering! Both for mother and baby, the mental and developmental benefits associated with breastfeeding are very important.

Recommendations for Breastfeeding Support from Surgeon General

Regina Benjamin, the Surgeon General under President Obama, put forth "The Surgeon General's Call to Action to Support Breastfeeding" in 2011. This was the first recognition from our government regarding the issue of the importance of breastfeeding and the need for its promotion and support in the US. The report highlighted the problems and barriers to the practice of breastfeeding in America and made 20 specific recommendations to reduce those barriers and promote and support breastfeeding. The 20 recommendations are as follows:

Action 1: SUPPORT MOTHERS: Give mothers the support they need to breastfeed their babies.

Action 2: FATHERS AND GRANDMOTHERS: Develop programs to educate fathers and grandmothers about breastfeeding.

Action 3: PEER COUNSELING: Strengthen programs that provide mother-to-mother support and peer counseling.

Action 4: COMMUNITY ORGANIZATIONS: Use community-based organizations to promote and support breastfeeding.

Action 5: PROMOTION CAMPAIGNS: Create a national campaign to promote breastfeeding.

Action 6: FORMULA MARKETING: Ensure that the marketing of infant formula is conducted in a way that minimizes its negative impacts on exclusive breastfeeding. Ideally, adopt "the Code" in America.

Action 7: MATERNITY CARE PRACTICES: Ensure that maternity care practices throughout the United States are fully supportive of breastfeeding. Baby-Friendly Hospital Initiative should be expanded to all birthing hospitals.

Action 8: CONTINUITY AND CARE: Develop systems to guarantee continuity of skilled support for lactation between hospitals and health care settings in the community (meaning, we need lactation consultants in outpatient care also).

Action 9: HEALTH CARE PROFESSIONAL TRAINING: Provide education and training in breastfeeding for all health professionals who care for women and children: nurses, doctors, midwives, nurse practitioners, physician assistants, dieticians, mental health care professionals, pharmacists, etcetera.

Action 10: STANDARD OF CARE: Include basic support for breastfeeding as a standard of care for midwives, obstetricians, family physicians, nurse practitioners, and pediatricians.

Action 11: ACCESS TO PROFESSIONAL CARE: Ensure access to services provided by International Board Certified Lactation Consultants. Increase number of lactation consultants, educational/clinical programs, and funding for the training/certification to meet this need for lactation consultants.

Action 12: DONOR MILK: Identify and address obstacles to greater availability of safe banked donor milk for fragile infants. Expand banked human milk access and funding for more human milk banks in the US.

Action 13: PAID LEAVE: Work toward establishing paid maternity/family leave for all employed mothers/families.

Action 14: WORKPLACE SUPPORT: Ensure that employers establish and maintain comprehensive, high-quality lactation support programs for their employees.

Action 15: BABIES AT WORK: Expand the use of programs in the workplace that allow lactating mothers to have direct access to their babies (during work hours).

Action 16: CHILD CARE: Ensure that all child care providers accommodate the needs of breastfeeding mothers and infants.

Action 17: RESEARCH FUNDING: Increase funding of high-quality research on breastfeeding.

Action 18: RESEARCH CAPACITY: Strengthen existing capacity and develop future capacity for conducting research on breastfeeding.

Action 19: NATIONAL MONITORING SYSTEM: Develop a national monitoring system to improve the tracking of breastfeeding rates as well as the policies and environmental factors that affect breastfeeding. This resulted in the Breastfeeding Report Card, but this needs improvement as noted in the first chapter.

Action 20: NATIONAL LEADERSHIP: Improve national leadership on the promotion and support of breastfeeding.

Most of these recommendations still are not anywhere near being realized, even though they were issued in 2011. Many barriers to breastfeeding still exist, and much needs to be done in the US to reach our national breastfeeding goals and adequately support breastfeeding mothers and babies for physical and mental health and well-being. These recommendations in the "Call to Action to Support Breastfeeding" need to be attended to, enacted, and expanded to cover even more breastfeeding barriers that were not addressed in this document! I am going to discuss some of the barriers that are causing substantial impediments to successful breastfeeding.

Excessive Medical Separation

Many babies are separated from their mothers after birth due to prematurity, difficult and prolonged medicalized births with poor <u>Apgar scores</u>, and other medical reasons. This separation of mom and baby is, of course, a big problem for breastfeeding. Moms separated from their babies suffer a delay in the stimulation of the breasts, which results in low production of milk. Even though many moms are encouraged to pump, pumping is not nearly as effective as breastfeeding in stimulating a milk supply. Added to this are the medical interventions that almost always accompany a high-risk or difficult birth, which cause a delay in milk production and can lead to anxiety and/or PPD.

At times, these medical separations are unavoidable due to extreme prematurity or other medical issues. However, hospital policies overuse this practice of high-risk, premature, and medically vulnerable babies going to <u>neonatal intensive care units (NICUs)</u> for closer monitoring. Doctors have valid concerns about high-risk babies and don't want to risk being sued if a baby has unmet medical needs, so they tend to have the high-risk baby go to NICU even if there is no acute medical need at the time. "Near-term" babies (babies born between 34 and 38 weeks gestation) are often sent to the NICU for the extra medical monitoring. Hospitals earn more money from using more medical interventions during births and babies going to the NICUs, so that is also an incentive for babies being separated from their mothers, since obstetrics (OB) care is a money loser for hospitals. Yes, some babies do need medical/NICU care, but many are sent there too readily and kept too long. NICU admission and separation from the breastfeeding mother is a recipe for breastfeeding cessation, which is not a good situation since the protections of breastfeeding are even more needed by these more vulnerable babies.

Kangaroo Care

On the other hand, if a more primary care approach to these vulnerable babies were used, it would include early and more intensive breastfeeding/lactation support and kangaroo care, keeping the breastfeeding mother and baby in close contact. If their breastfeeding needs/problems would have been quickly identified and given attention and support immediately, their feeding and temperature problems might have been managed without the baby going to the NICU and being separated from their mothers.

Breastfeeding and skin-to-skin care (or kangaroo care) are utilized much more often in other countries than in the US and avoids the separation of mom and baby. This kangaroo care, of course, involves breastfeeding management and support as an integral part of the management of fragile babies. We need more hospitals that practice and support kangaroo care, and we need more IBCLCs for these fragile babies, instead of separating them from their moms, medicalizing their care, and causing anxious and rough starts to their lives as families!

Overreliance on Weight Gain as Indicator of Need for Supplemental Formula

There are other ways our medical care system (both hospital and outpatient care) mismanages breastfeeding mothers and babies and thwarts their efforts to breastfeed. Examples are the overreliance on weight gain as the main parameter used to assess adequacy of breastfeeding. This is a problem especially because the overuse of IV fluids causes babies to be overhydrated in labor and delivery and to subsequently lose more fluid weight as a result. Medical policies state that babies who lose more than 10% of their birth weight need supplementation. This leads to doctors prescribing formula to supplement the breastfed baby who has lost too much weight. This early formula use is also most often prescribed without a prior order for a lactation consultant to be called in to assess and give breastfeeding support and to help mend the breastfeeding problem before the application of the "Band-Aid" of formula supplementation.

Early formula usage is especially detrimental to breastfeeding success because the supplemented baby feeds less often at the breast, causing a delay in milk production, and because it threatens a mom's confidence in her breastfeeding ability. The unaddressed breastfeeding problem then becomes a greater problem, causing much maternal anxiety and requiring huge efforts to correct. Moms are often told to breastfeed, pump after each breastfeed, and supplement (which is called triple feeding). Even when breastfeeding is going well, it is a full-time job of eight to 10 hours per day during the early weeks. Mothers breastfeeding/pumping/supplementing are spending upwards of 20 hours per day on this triple-feeding medical regimen. This causes lack of sleep and is a major factor in postpartum depression, anxiety, problems bonding with the baby, and, sadly, not being able to enjoy being a mother! No wonder so many mothers give up on breastfeeding!

Often a doctor will order two ounces of formula to supplement (for the baby with a slow weight gain) after each breastfeed, which is *fully formula feeding* since a normal full bottle-feeding amount for a newborn is two ounces. This makes the baby not be motivated to breastfeed effectively, to prefer the fast-flowing bottle feeds, and to reject breastfeeding. Then the lack of frequent and adequate breastfeeds leads to the loss of the mother's milk production since milk production is a demand-based system. After moms leave the hospital, they are often not given the services of lactation professionals to address the breastfeeding problems because few pediatric offices have lactation professionals in their practice. Independent outpatient lactation services are lacking in most communities. This lack of access to lactation services unfortunately happens when many mothers experience engorgement and are at the *greatest need for breastfeeding support*. Many moms/families do not have the family support and financial ability to seek the services of a distant lactation consultant on their own, and even if they did, with all the time they are spending breastfeeding, pumping, and supplementing, they don't have the energy or time to schedule another appointment with another provider! It sure would be nice if our health/medical care system recognized the need for lactation consultants to be an integral part of our outpatient pediatric care system! Lactation services can also be delivered as part of home-based care, but there are few lactation professionals working in that capacity due to too few lactation professionals, problems getting insurance reimbursement, and licensing issues for this still young profession.

Some mothers and babies have even been reported to the Division of Family Services (DFS) for refusing to supplement (knowing that all the supplementation will cause breastfeeding problems and not feeling it is necessary) when their baby was medically diagnosed with slow weight gain. Many breastfed babies with slow weight gain are misdiagnosed with "failure to thrive," which is considered a medical emergency. Failure to thrive is overdiagnosed due to heavy reliance on weight gain as the only parameter of breastfeeding adequacy. Many other parameters of breastfeeding adequacy should be considered, like frequency of pees and poops, softening of a mother's breast after a breastfeed, baby's contentment after a breastfeed, and a good milk transfer as observed by a lactation professional. However, these other parameters are most often not considered before a breastfeeding baby is diagnosed with failure to thrive and prescribed heavy formula supplementation! Sadly, most babies diagnosed with slow weight gain never get to see a lactation consultant for a thorough breastfeeding assessment before they are recommended to start supplemental formula. This amounts to a form of medical neglect that would not exist if breastfeeding was not so undervalued in our country.

Lactation Hospital Staffing Issues

Although there are International Board Certified Lactation Consultants (IBCLCs) on staff at hospitals, there are far too few, and they are not called in often or soon enough when needed. Lactation care for high-risk mothers and babies is time and care intensive; I remember needing to spend more than one hour with many moms and newborns who were having breastfeeding difficulties and revisiting them more than once in my work shift. But hospital IBCLCs often have over 20 mother/baby clients that they need to visit in their eight-hour work shift due to unrecognized understaffing for lactation services! Many hospital IBCLCs have to cover both the postpartum services and the NICUs. Some hospitals also require the IBCLCs to cover outpatient and employee lactation services as well. This means that lactation services are spread way too thin, and if the IBCLC is working with high-need babies and mothers, they don't have time to spend with others.

The hospital or medical care system usually sees lactation services as less essential or incidental and does not recognize the importance of well-staffed, easily accessible lactation services for all breastfeeding mothers and babies. For example, many hospital lactation services only serve breastfeeding mothers and babies who have an order written by an MD for their services as a way to limit the demand and work for their too few numbers of lactation professionals employed at that hospital. Breastfeeding is a primary and essential form of public health and should not need a "tertiary care" RX for the attainment of these basic health services. Also, comparatively, lactation professional-to-client ratios are way too high, as mentioned before, with staff IBCLCs serving as many as 20 clients simultaneously. Compare this to RNs working in labor and delivery who have a recommended one to three clients because it is recognized that laboring clients need intensive care. Breastfeeding support is less intensive than childbirth but more intensive than other types of care—yet the IBCLC-to-client ratio is too large, as noted above. If all RNs working in labor and delivery and postpartum services were also certified as IBCLCs, this would greatly help to solve the problem of understaffed lactation services. Then the other IBCLCs could be staffed separately for the NICUs, outpatient lactation needs, and hospital breastfeeding employee services. Expanding the Baby-Friendly program to all birthing hospitals to support all labor and delivery staff to become trained and certified as IBCLCs would allow all mothers and babies to be served as they need and deserve.

Need for More Lactation Professionals

In 2019, there were 17,417 IBCLCs in America, and we had approximately 3.8 million babies born in America, so that means there is approximately one active IBCLC for every 218 babies born per year. Not all mothers will have the need of lactation services, but others will need lactation services many times throughout the course of their breastfeeding relationship. So "IBCLC per birth" is not an ideal metric. We need to factor in the average length of breastfeeding in days and months as it relates to the need for lactation services. We also need to figure in our national breastfeeding goals as to how many lactation professionals are needed in America. It would be wise to increase the number of IBCLCs to promote breastfeeding and get national breastfeeding rates up, just like a company would hire more salespeople to increase the sales of their product. I realize that IBCLCs don't make hospitals money, but they save many medical care dollars in the long run!

We clearly need more qualified lactation consultants working with newborn (birth to 3 months) babies and their mothers, as that is when the need is greatest for lactation services. We especially need more IBCLCs working in hospitals and in communities where there are high rates of prematurity, infant mortality, and other high-risk neonatal issues. We need IBCLCs and certified lactation counselors (CLCs) for outpatient and pediatric services also, as breastfeeding problems can occur after the mother and baby have left the birthing hospital! It would certainly help if there was universal insurance payment for lactation services so that new families with the extra expenses of a new baby did not have to pay out of pocket for lactation services.

States with a higher number of breastfeeding service providers and support groups enjoy higher breastfeeding rates. When there have been shortages of other health care professionals, government funding to educate/train more of those needed professionals has been made available to offset those shortages. We need government funding to address the shortage of IBCLCs in the US and insurance-covered payment for IBCLC services to help moms and babies get the care they need as well as to entice people into a profession that adequately compensates its breastfeeding practitioners. We also need more universities to establish in-house educational lactation programs at the university level instead of the current situation that forces people who are interested in gaining certification to do it independently of a university program. I have known many who have had trouble getting the clinical hours they need to sit for the IBCLC exam due to not having established lactation programs at the university level that affiliates with a clinical setting.

Our current mishmash of health insurance policies and coverage is also confusing regarding what and how insurance covers breastfeeding needs. Most moms must pay an outpatient IBCLC out of pocket and then seek reimbursement for those costs (like she needs the extra work!). A typical cost for a comprehensive IBCLC appointment can range from $150 to $300. Keep in mind that highly trained IBCLCs typically spend a couple of hours doing a thorough breastfeeding observation and assessment, pre- and post-breastfeeding weights, breast-/nipple-care assessment, education, product use explanation, pumping assessment, and breastfeeding teaching. Charting, communicating with an MD as needed, referrals, and follow-up calls take extra time. IBCLCs are underpaid for the intensive care they give. Yet it is quite expensive and hard to become an IBCLC, requiring many hours of specialized breastfeeding seminars and clinical hours and an expensive exam to become certified to practice as an IBCLC. This hardship and expense to become an IBCLC, coupled with the inadequate compensation, add up to another bad recipe for breastfeeding support. We desperately need more government funding for lactation education and programs to get more lactation professionals certified.

A need for more Certified Lactation Counselors (CLCs) also exists, as they are valuable in their roles supporting breastfeeding mothers and babies in community settings. The certification process for a CLC is shorter and easier and less intensive, but they are not usually considered qualified to work in the health care setting. Many IBCLCs use the CLC training and experience as a step to becoming certified as an IBCLC. More of both types of lactation professionals are needed! Information about where to access the qualifications and certification for both is listed in the Notes at the end of this book.

Our unmet need for more CLCs and IBCLCs is another example of how our lack of breastfeeding data perpetuates a lack of lactation professionals and good policies to support breastfeeding by not accurately documenting the need for them.

We also could use more diversity and expanded access to other community breastfeeding supporters such as La Leche League Leaders, Black Mothers' Breastfeeding Association, Breastfeeding USA Counselors, I AM: Breastfeeding, and others. Mothers who have more paid time off from work can more easily make use of these free community breastfeeding resources.

Summary

To summarize this chapter, I have discussed the developmental, mental, and neuroprotective benefits of breastfeeding, especially direct breastfeeding versus bottle-feeding pumped milk. Next I reviewed the good but unrealized "Action to Support Breastfeeding" put forth by Surgeon General Regina Benjamin in 2011. The issues of medical separation of mothers and newborns with medical complications and the overreliance on newborn weight gain as the main indicator of feeding adequacy, causing greater use of supplemental formula, are a recipe for breastfeeding failure. These medically fragile babies, who already have health problems, don't need additional health problems related to breastfeeding failure. We need earlier and more intensive breastfeeding support for these most vulnerable babies and their mothers, and we need more accessible lactation services and more—and more diverse—certified lactation consultants. The ingredients of breastfeeding support covered in this chapter are to prioritize and support the process of *direct breastfeeding* rather than *breast milk feeding*; to follow through on the 20 recommendations in the "Call to Action to Support Breastfeeding;" have more lactation support for the breastfeeding issues of fragile babies, keeping mothers and babies together as much as possible; and get more lactation professionals trained and certified to meet the growing demand and to help attain our national breastfeeding goals.

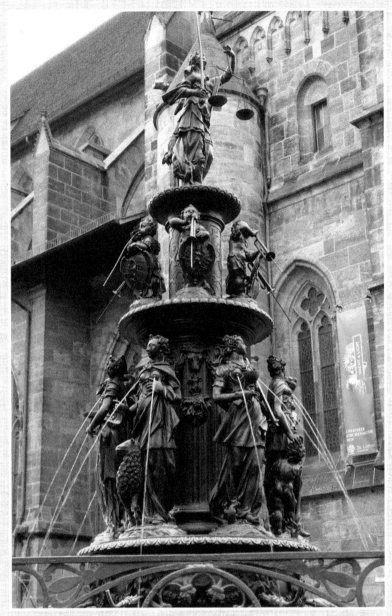

The Tugendbrunnen (Fountain of Virtues) in Nuremberg features representations of the virtues, crowned by the figure of Justice. The virtues are Justice, Temperance, Fortitude, Patience, Faith, Hope, and Charity. The statue's sculptor, Benedikt Wurzelbauer (1548–1620), used mother's milk to represent these virtues. This statue indicates how a mother's milk is not only good for an individual baby but is also a social good.

— 3 —

Gender, Work, Racial, and Health Equity

We are not reaching all of our national (or personal) breastfeeding goals in the US, and that causes us to not reach our other national health-related goals. It also causes a lot of <u>health inequities</u>, health care inequities, gender inequities, and social inequities. Breastfeeding is promoted and encouraged by our government, health care providers, and institutions but is not accurately counted or adequately supported. This leads to the situation where women are left to shoulder all the responsibility of breastfeeding and suffer from the disappointment, regret, and guilt of not meeting their breastfeeding goals. This is a systemic failure inflicted upon America's mothers—and a form of gender discrimination.

Because we lack national paid family leave, most working mothers are forced to return to paying work before breastfeeding is well established. Women make up around half of the American workforce. Less than one-fourth of working mothers receive any paid family leave, and if they do, it usually only lasts six to 12 weeks. A woman reentering employment soon after a birth is three times more likely to stop breastfeeding sooner than intended compared to the mother who has extended time off. Mothers who decide to give up their jobs to stay at home with their young baby lose their place on the career ladder and all the benefits that go with being gainfully employed.

Low-income mothers, single mothers, mothers working without any paid leave and in non-breastfeeding-friendly work situations have many additional barriers to breastfeeding. Most of the mothers I see in <u>Women, Infants, and Children (WIC)</u> return to work much earlier due to financial need. This much-earlier return to work, which is often not breastfeeding-friendly, is a huge barrier to breastfeeding. I hear about their struggles in my work in a WIC center, and the lower WIC breastfeeding rates reflect their struggles. In 2018, WIC reported national breastfeeding rates of only 32.4% (12.5% of infants were fully breastfed and 19.9% were partially breastfed). More about WIC is discussed in the next chapter.

The lack of comprehensive national health insurance is another breastfeeding barrier for many American mothers. Insurance coverage is a huge expense for American companies, and consequently, many employers avoid paying for health insurance by hiring part-time workers who don't qualify for health insurance benefits. Low-income and part-time working breastfeeding mothers are especially affected by this practice. Even if they have Medicaid coverage for their pregnancies, they are kicked off six weeks after giving birth (right after their postpartum appointment). The low-income family can get Medicaid for the baby, but in states that have not expanded Medicaid coverage, the mother cannot get Medicaid coverage. Keeping a mother healthy is important for her baby's well-being, but lack of medical insurance forces many mothers to forgo needed health care. It's sad that a mother's health is so undervalued in this country that she has to forgo health insurance and subsequently go without health care and breastfeeding support if she cannot afford it!

American mothers who have private/employer-sponsored health insurance must return to work to keep their health insurance because their medical insurance is attached to their employment status. Even if they could afford to stay home for longer, they must return to work to maintain health insurance coverage or pay for costly private medical insurance. Breastfeeding is recommended for a year or more, and breastfeeding mothers can have medical needs related to breastfeeding, so continued health insurance coverage is needed! A national paid leave and national health insurance coverage go hand in hand with breastfeeding support.

The Work and Time of Breastfeeding

In my many years of work, I have often heard, "Breastfeeding takes so much time," from moms who are struggling to go back to work outside the home while managing a family and homestead on top of breastfeeding a young baby. **I agree: breastfeeding *does* take time, effort, and energy!** Many think of breastfeeding in a sentimental way, as a mom sitting and relaxing with her baby, taking a break from work, being waited upon by others—that is NOT the case for most breastfeeding moms! Or, if a mom does receive that kind of support, it is only for a short time in the immediate period after birth!

When a mom is fully/exclusively breastfeeding a young baby, breastfeeding, by itself, is more than a full-time job! It takes an average of seven to 10 hours per day in *actual* feeding time with a new baby if breastfeeding is going well! When mothers are having breastfeeding difficulties, they might be spending many more hours in a day on breastfeeding, pumping, or bottle or alternative feeding and going for pediatric appointments and weight checks. Later, breastfeeding gets easier, more convenient, and less time consuming, but for the first months of breastfeeding, to keep the milk flowing, producing, and growing for her rapidly growing baby, a mom needs to breastfeed an average of eight to 12 times per day (or more often during growth spurts). Those frequent breastfeedings add up in time expenditure but are much needed for establishing a mother's milk production. *Yes, breastfeeding and caring for a young baby is much more than a full-time job!*

Breastfeeding does take a lot of time, but that also means that the baby gets to spend more time in mom's loving and nurturing arms! Feeding directly from the breast means getting a lot of neurocognitive, sensory-rich stimulation and loving attention from being so close to a vested person—mom! This is in addition to the best nutrition and immune protection of their own mother's milk made especially suited to their needs! Breastfeeding is so much more than just milk or basic nutrition! Breastfeeding is as much of a *process* as it is a product, and many of its benefits come from the process of breastfeeding, which takes a mother's time. America's focus on *breast milk* instead of *breastfeeding* ignores the rich experience and productiveness of direct breastfeeding that is so important to breastfeeding success.

Direct breastfeeding needs time to become well established and is a learned process for the mother and newborn. Direct breastfeeding is also important for keeping a mother's milk production ample and transfers greater protection to the baby than pumped milk feeding. For breastfeeding success and a good milk supply, it is recommended to focus on direct breastfeeding and avoid bottles in the early weeks. That means that feeding the baby is solely mom's responsibility, and she can't be separated from her infant for long until they are taking a bottle well from others.

How Returning to Work Interferes with Breastfeeding

Sadly, moms who return to work early tend to focus on pumping breast milk to get a "stash" of breast milk started rather than focusing on direct breastfeeding. This takes more time away from baby and breastfeeding. Pumping takes more time and effort to do, involves extra cleanup and storage, yet pumping usually doesn't stimulate a mother's milk production as well as direct breastfeeding does. Mothers who have to do a lot of pumping for breast milk/bottle feeds often lose their milk supply much sooner, or they get so tired of pumping, they give it up.

Also, a common breastfeeding difficulty arises when babies get introduced to bottles too early and often and start preferring the fast, easy-flowing bottle and rejecting the work of direct breastfeeding. A less common problem is some breastfed babies don't like bottles and refuse them even if introduced at a reasonable time. I've known babies who refused to take a feed until their mom returned from work. This puts them at risk for losing weight and also stresses the breastfeeding mother, knowing that her baby is hungry and waiting for her to get home from work to feed!

Working necessitates the separation of mother and baby for a substantial time of each working day, which makes it necessary for a mother to pump her milk while at work or she will lose her milk production. When a mother returns to work while her young baby is exclusively breastfeeding and going through frequent growth spurts, she needs to pump more often than every four hours to keep her milk supply ample to meet her growing child's needs. Since the current pumping break law is tied to the work break of 15 minutes every 4 hours, this is inadequate for mothers trying to keep up their milk supply. I have heard from so many mothers who get too busy at work to pump as often as they need to. Then the less-frequent pumping schedule causes them to have too little milk production for their baby's needs. Pumping itself also does not stimulate a mother's milk production as effectively as direct breastfeeding does. Direct breastfeeding involves the movement of the baby's jaw, the tongue movements, and suction. Pumping is suction only, so it is not as effective as the baby at extracting the milk. Milk removal is what stimulates more milk to be produced, and when a breastfeeding mother lets her breasts stay full, she lowers her milk production. Unrelieved breast fullness also puts a mother at risk for plugged ducts and breast infections. This is the reason that working mothers not able to directly breastfeed their babies for a large part of their day during full-time work hours tend to lose their milk supply and wean sooner than mothers who are able to do mostly direct breastfeeding.

Pumping at work also causes the working mother more stress, as she must use *all her break and lunch time for pumping* and has less time for relaxation, which is so important! Sometimes the baby who gets a lot of bottles while a mother works starts to prefer the fast, easy flow of the bottles and starts refusing to breastfeed when the mother is home. These hardships are all a part of the slippery slope to the loss of her milk production/supply and an earlier-than-intended weaning with less dose-related benefits. This is well documented by research and the fact that two-thirds of American mothers are not meeting their breastfeeding goals: only 36% are still breastfeeding at the end of one year, down from an 84% initiation rate. So free, insurance-provided breast pumps and pumping time allowed on a mother's break time are not effective at helping moms to breastfeed for the recommended time of a year or more. An analogy to the issue of pumping at work versus receiving paid leave is like wearing face masks to avoid air pollution instead of addressing the air pollution—basically, a "Band-Aid solution." As noted in Chapter 2, the act of breastfeeding is so much more than just nutrition for a baby. Extra time to stay at home with a baby to get breastfeeding well established with paid leave and health care coverage is what mothers really need.

Breastfeeding Barriers and Racial Inequities

African American mothers unfortunately experience many more breastfeeding barriers and consequently have the lowest breastfeeding rates in the US. According to the CDC, Black mothers struggle with breastfeeding because they return earlier to work, have less economic security/suffer from greater poverty, have higher rates of single parenthood, receive less information/education about the importance of breastfeeding from their health care providers, and have less access to professional and community breastfeeding support. Many of my African American pregnant clients report that no one else in their family has breastfed, and because of this, they have less support from their families. There is a paucity of lactation professionals who are Black and serve in Black communities.

Unfortunately, African American babies also experience the highest premature and medically complicated birth rates, which make breastfeeding more difficult but also *more important* for avoiding related life-threatening illnesses. African American maternal and infant mortality rates are the highest rates in the US—sometimes three times higher in some Black communities than the average infant mortality rate! African American mothers also have higher rates of pre-eclampsia, obesity, and metabolic disease, all causing more problems with childbirth and breastfeeding. African American mothers unfortunately experience more medical interventions in their childbirths due to these medical conditions. A medicalized childbirth often results in the mothers and babies being separated due to babies needing to go to the NICU. This higher rate of medical interventions in childbirth often leads to more problems with breastfeeding right from the start, as discussed in the previous chapter. These breastfeeding problems associated with medical issues often result in a much earlier than intended weaning to formula feeding. So, these Black mothers and babies, who are *most at risk* for higher morbidity and mortality due to medical issues, have the *least support* and success with breastfeeding. This situation of having more medical problems coupled with less breastfeeding support causes them to be medically entrenched due to higher rates of illness associated with lower breastfeeding success. Social inequities are also greater due to poor health and the subsequent need for more time, energy, and family resources to be spent on medical care. This bad recipe leads to greater rates of lifelong illnesses for Black mothers and babies, and it is a serious and untreated health inequity.

America protects fetuses, but as soon as the baby is born, we let the moms and babies fend for themselves through our lack of breastfeeding services, paid family leave, and comprehensive health coverage. Medical companies profit from our lack of breastfeeding support in the short term and the long term. When parents can't breastfeed their babies, they must purchase products and services such as formula, bottles, and medicines. Then, the illnesses that result from breastfeeding failures line the pockets of the rich medical industries in America and leave mothers feeling sad and abandoned. This is well documented in Kimberly Seals Allers' well-named book *The Big Letdown*!

Health, gender, racial, economic, and social inequities in the US would be lessened if *all* mothers received the paid time off work to get breastfeeding well established, support and resources that they need to overcome their breastfeeding and mothering challenges, and national health care coverage not dependent on return to employment! A national health insurance program goes hand in hand with a national paid leave program so parents raising children are not left uninsured as they do the work of caring and nurturing our most precious resources—our children.

Unbridled Formula Promotion in Low-Income and Black Communities

Unbridled formula promotion and frequent medical recommendations for formula supplementation is a big barrier to breastfeeding success among populations at risk. I have worked with so many mothers in WIC who experience these breastfeeding barriers and succumb to the temptation and all-too-common recommendations for early and heavy formula use as a Band-Aid solution (rather than receiving the needed lactation/breastfeeding support). It is a sad fact that low-income and Black mothers receive less breastfeeding education and referrals to lactation services and more frequent recommendations to use formula when there are breastfeeding challenges such as a baby's weight not increasing or newborn jaundice. (This, too, is addressed in *The Big Letdown*.) Formula is served up on a "silver platter" (or maybe I should say in a "silver bottle") in low-income and communities of color by the family and friends who did not breastfeed themselves, doctors' recommendations, WIC's free formula vouchers, grocery stores, and food pantries. This Band-Aid of supplemental formula usage causes mothers to lose their milk supply and wean much earlier than they intend. Weaning binds them to an expensive system of having to buy a costly but inferior product (formula) for their baby's survival. This is tragic because the benefits of breastfeeding are dose-related, and those who breastfeed for less time enjoy less health benefits.

A mother who weans earlier than intended from breastfeeding often experiences regret, sadness, and even guilt over not being able to meet her breastfeeding goals. Too little time to get breastfeeding and mothering off to a good start increases stress on mothers, leading to more postpartum anxiety and depression. Postpartum depression is becoming more common, and the stress of returning to work too early, leaving your newborn, and worrying about feeding/pumping increase the risk of postpartum depression. Breastfeeding problems increase the risk of postpartum depression, *yet breastfeeding success decreases the risk of postpartum depression.* Many cases of postpartum depression could be avoided if mothers received more time off work and better support, which they need and deserve! Mothers could relax and enjoy the work of breastfeeding so much more if they didn't have to work another full-time job that takes them away from their baby, spend all their work break time pumping milk, and keep up with all the other work they do to keep a family and home running.

The following notes (all from mothers I have worked with through WIC) exemplify their worries and regrets about returning to work, using formula, and losing their milk supply:

Mom #1 was interested in breastfeeding. She did not breastfeed her others due to returning to work, but she wouldn't be returning to work after this baby was born. She said she didn't feel breastfeeding while working was possible, and she was sorry she didn't try with her first baby.

Mom #2 was planning on weaning from breastfeeding due to returning to work. Pumping was too time-consuming, she stated, and she couldn't take regular breaks to pump in her job. She planned to wean by our next appointment and wanted to get more formula to supplement.

Mom #3 was mostly breastfeeding with her baby and stated she breastfed around four times per 24 hours, pumped six times per 24 hours, and got four ounces each time she pumped. She gave some formula also, she stated, even though she has enough expressed breast milk, as she wanted her baby to get used to the taste of formula, since she worried she would eventually not have enough expressed breast milk. She was returning to full-time school and a weekend job soon and would be separated from her baby often. She wanted to save some of her expressed breast milk for later so he would have some continued immune protection after she lost her milk supply, she stated.

Mom #4 is breastfeeding with her baby but stated she couldn't pump any milk at all and she had tried different pumps. She was worried about returning to work and wanted to start her stash of expressed breast milk.

Mom #5 stated she went back to full-time work, and although she received a double electric pump from her insurance company, she couldn't pump enough milk for her baby. She started supplementing with formula at one month of age, then her baby started to get fussy at breastfeeds and refused to breastfeed after getting regular bottles. She lost her milk supply and had to wean to complete formula feeding when he was two months old. She stated she was disappointed, as her breastfeeding goal was for six months. She said working and breastfeeding was a lot harder than she thought it would be.

Mom #6 was currently fully breastfeeding and stated her baby did not like bottles, so she is worried about her baby going hungry at day care because he refuses bottles.

Mom #7 continued to fully breastfeed and stated she loved breastfeeding but had concerns about pumping enough milk when she returned to work. She worried that she wouldn't have time for pumping at work and wanted to have plenty of pumped milk stored up before she returned to work. She had lots of worries about her milk supply.

Mom #8 was fully breastfeeding her baby. Her baby was not accepting bottles yet. We discussed her return to work, and she stated she was fearful of her baby being fussy and crying when she was gone, as well as the day care workers being abusive because her baby was fussy.

Mom #9 was trying to re-lactate but had been working a lot and was separated from her baby. She stated, "I know it is important to breastfeed, but now my baby is refusing to stay at breast for a feed. I guess she prefers the bottle/formula now because she gets so many of them, since I have been working a lot of hours."

Mom #10 is partially breastfeeding with her baby and complained of lots of stress, restarting smoking, and going back to work as reasons for no longer exclusively breastfeeding. She breastfeeds at night and formula feeds in daytime. She states baby still prefers to breastfeed, and she feels bad about giving bottles, but she read that she should wait two hours after smoking a cigarette to breastfeed, and so she does not breastfeed often. She also is working a lot of hours to catch up after being off from work after giving birth. Weaning from breastfeeding is a greater risk for ill health than baby getting exposed to cigarettes via breastfeeding, so I encouraged her to go ahead and breastfeed even if she can't quit smoking.

These notes show the difficulties, concerns, fears, and disappointments that so many WIC-dependent mothers experience as they to return to work outside the home when their young babies are still breastfeeding frequently and fully reliant on breastfeeding for all their nutrition. The low-income, single-parent, and African American mothers I work with in WIC return to work so much earlier than others due to financial needs. They don't have the time and resources to seek and receive lactation services for any breastfeeding problems they experience. In addition, they often don't even get paid sick time or vacation, so any time they take off after the birth of a baby is causing them financial stress. This sad fact, coupled with their higher rates of medical and social risks due to being impoverished, is a very bad recipe indeed!

Time, Recognition, and Support Needed for Mothering

The fact that the work of bearing, birthing, and breastfeeding our progeny—the work of continuing and nurturing the human race—is not "counted" and given recognition as part of our economy is one big symptom of how women are taken advantage of in our patriarchal society. Why isn't breastfeeding considered as part of our gross domestic product (GDP)? Marilyn French, in her book *The War Against Women*, points out that all or most of the burden of nurturing and raising children is on women, but that this burden is not recognized or rewarded as work. Breastfeeding is a prime example of this unrecognized work! She states this lack of recognition and reward for this necessary and worthy work is systemic discrimination against women and is a major reason for the disadvantaged situation women endure in America, earning an average of 79% of what men earn for similar work.

American mothers who do leave their careers to be a stay-at-home mother incur a loss of status on the career ladder while they are dedicating themselves to raising the most important asset— our children and future workers/citizens. This demonstrates a fundamental example of **gender discrimination** in America! American mothers' breastfeeding efforts and mothering work are not even being counted, much less given credence by our economic system.

Our children are the future citizens and workers of America, and our precious mothers are the ones who bear, birth, and breastfeed them! Recognition of the work of mothering and breastfeeding is desperately needed in our country. National paid family leave legislation would help mothers both be successful and have time to enjoy breastfeeding and mothering! It would also help to compensate mothers for their gender-related work of mothering and breastfeeding. Increasing the number of mothers who breastfeed, and for longer duration, would reduce the incidence of costly illnesses and would, therefore, save health care dollars that could offset costs of a national paid family leave. Ideally, more paid leave time could accrue as we monitor the success of the program and the dollars saved in other health/medical care costs over time. This paid leave issue has been addressed many times in the past but has never received commitment from our *national* government to make it happen. Maybe this is the reason many families are having smaller families or choosing not to have children at all!

A Birth Strike in America for Paid Leave

American women are having fewer babies. This is good, as we need to slow our birth rate due to overpopulation concerns, with projections that we will have 9 to 10 billion people on earth by 2050, but slowing it too fast can cause problems in the working-to-nonworking population ratio. The population of our country is already getting significantly older, with projections that one out of five Americans will be over 65 years of age and will outnumber the young by 2030. That leaves fewer working-age adults to support both young and old.

Many women are choosing not to have babies or to have fewer babies due to the lack of paid leave and lack of support in America for family life and the financial struggles associated with having children. The US now has the slowest growth rate in a century due to fewer births, increasing deaths as our population ages, and less immigration due to the recent restrictions. Also, many women are experiencing fertility problems due to obesity, diabetes, and metabolic syndrome (in part due to the low breastfeeding rates of the 20th century). The 2018 CDC birth rate was 1.73, which is a record low for the US.

Women in America can use this issue of lower birth rates as a calling card to gain paid leave and more support for breastfeeding and parenting because America needs babies, and only women have that ability to bear, birth, and breastfeed babies! This has been the case in many other countries in response to falling birth rates. In some countries, women/families receive not only lengthy paid parental leave after the birth of a child, but also childcare and preschool funding, monthly allowances, and bonuses for children born! This is well documented in a new book called *Birth Strike: The Hidden Fight Over Women's Work*, by Jenny Brown, a leader in the National Women's Liberation.

American women could use their fertility to leverage paid leave and other rights needed to do the work of nurturing young babies—the future workers of our country. A *coordinated* and *advertised* American birth strike could be arranged through social and traditional media, and if even 30% of American women participated and *made it known* that this is what they are doing, it would send a powerful message: NO PAID LEAVE, NO BABIES! It is actually already happening, so why not use this fact of lowering birth rates in the US to advance the issue of paid leave?

Recommendations for National Six-Month Paid Family Leave

The US is the wealthiest country and the only large industrialized country to never institute a national policy for paid family leave. America has left the issue of paid leave up to employers to give, or not, paid leave as a "benefit" of their job. This way of American thinking mislabels what should be a right as an arbitrary benefit. We do this with health care coverage also—it's a benefit from employers instead of a right.

Currently, fewer than one-quarter of American families receive any paid leave benefits after the birth of a baby through their employer, and it is usually only for six to 12 weeks. The Family and Medical Leave Act (FMLA) of 1993 only guarantees unpaid leave, which is also unfair. Having a baby causes greater financial needs, and with 47% of mothers as the sole earners for their families, taking unpaid leave is too great a financial hardship, and consequently, is not utilized by many. Most American families must use all their sick and vacation time to take any time off or to increase the paltry post-birth leave of six to 12 weeks (if they have that benefit). Then, when the new mother or father needs sick leave or wants vacation time, they don't have any left until it accrues again. How awful America treats its new parents and babies!

The Obama administration proposed the FAMILY Act, a national paid family and medical leave program, but it did not gain support from Congress and sadly was not passed into law. Instead, the Obama administration achieved insurance coverage of pumps through the Affordable Care Act (ACA); passed the Break Time for Nursing Mothers law, which covers pumping breaks for hourly workers; and publicized Surgeon General Regina Benjamin's 2011 "Call to Action to Support Breastfeeding," a plan for greater breastfeeding support in America. This legislation and coverage for pumping at work and getting free pumps from insurance is like going through the back door, or a fringe type of solution. A national paid leave would be a front door or primary solution for breastfeeding support; however, Congress and corporate America would not, did not, and still have not made that a reality.

The comedian John Oliver did a very apropos commentary on this subject for Mother's Day, quoted in *Mother Jones* magazine by Inae Oh:

"This is not how it's supposed to work," Oliver said. "Mothers shouldn't have to stitch together time to recover from childbirth the same way that we plan a four-day weekend in Atlantic City." Much of this problem is two-fold, Oliver explains, with companies refusing to offer paid leave packages and fearmongering lawmakers claiming any federal mandates to do so would only hurt businesses. "You can't go on and on about how much you love moms but fail to pass legislation that makes life easier for them."

President Trump's empty promise of six weeks paid leave was much too little and was abandoned early in Trump's tenure. There are no current plans for a national paid family leave in the US. Congress has only just recently increased the family leave for military from six weeks to 12—but that is still too short and covers too few!

So, it is left up to the states, and only a few states have enacted any paid family leave policy: California, Washington, Rhode Island, New Jersey, and New York are the only states that cover paid leave for all their workers. Different states fund it in different manners, offering variable amounts of wage replacement and durations of paid time off, but none more than just 12 weeks. More states are planning to offer paid leave, but each state has a different plan/method for amount of time off, funding method, and wage coverage.

State-by-state and business-by-business methods of covering paid leave are way too confusing, complicated, and nonequitable. Leaving it up to businesses and corporations to give paid leave as a benefit results in a lot of variability and nonequitable distribution of benefits. Low-paid and part-time workers rarely get benefits such as vacation and sick days, much less any paid leave. This "corporate paid leave benefit" is not guaranteed as a nationally covered right. Some parents live in one state and work in another state or work at two or more different jobs—so which state law or business practice of paid leave would apply to them? Americans are too mobile and interconnected to not have a national plan for this important and *basic right* of paid family leave!

Keeping mothers home with a *national* paid family leave serves to recognize and validate the mothering role, which is so important to our national health and economy. *All* mothers and babies deserve paid leave **for at least six months** to get breastfeeding, infant care, bonding, and parenting off to the healthiest start. Since the recommendation is for exclusive breastfeeding until six months of age (when babies can start foods), paid leave should be at least for six months. The extra time at home will help mothers to breastfeed their babies for longer and for babies to receive more parental attention without another job competing for the mother's time and energy. We will all reap the benefits of healthier and less stressed children and mothers when we have a national paid leave! It will also go a long way to help lessen the health and social inequities experienced by lower-income, African American, single-parent, and immigrant mothers! More parents being home with babies on paid leave will also be good for communities as they will be more able to see what is going on in their communities and have time to participate in community activities.

Sometimes it might be the non-breastfeeding father or partner who stays home with the baby, and they support the breastfeeding mother by doing the caregiving, taking the baby to the mom at her job for a breastfeed at lunch or break time, and doing the home and family work. Then the breastfeeding mom can focus on breastfeeding when she gets home from work and not have to do extra work at home. Mothers (and fathers, partners, adoptive parents, and trans or "chest-feeding" parents of all kinds) deserve this paid family leave, as they are feeding and caring for the most vulnerable citizens of this world! That's why it needs to be a paid *family* leave—so *families* can decide what works best for them.

Mothers should not be forced into choosing between their motherhood role and their career or being overworked and stressed by trying to do both simultaneously! It's so sad that most American moms do not receive the support most other countries give to their mothers and children by allowing them to stay at home with their young babies and receive the needed financial support of a national paid family leave. This is a *gender inequity* that ignores motherhood as a social good. Mothers are bearing, birthing, and breastfeeding our future American workers—so why do we not have a comprehensive national paid family leave in America?! Because we ignore human capital in favor of monetary capital by allowing our **industry and government to get a free ride on the backs of American mothers when it comes to bearing, birthing, and breastfeeding our progeny.** A national paid family leave is one of the most important ways that our country can support breastfeeding mothers, babies, and families and, importantly, improve equality and health equity for all women, since they do the work of breastfeeding.

Comprehensive National Health Insurance—Medicare for All

American mothers who don't get health insurance from a working spouse must return to work too soon or pay very expensive prices to maintain their health insurance coverage through the Consolidated Omnibus Budget Reconciliation Act (COBRA). Since many American mothers are single and have financial insecurity, that means that this insurance coverage issue affects a lot of mothers. As I said before, even Medicaid coverage ends six to eight weeks postpartum. Babies need their mothers' care above and beyond the issue of breastfeeding, but this early return to work for the reason of insurance coverage is another breastfeeding barrier; those mothers do not have enough time to get breastfeeding firmly established. A comprehensive national health insurance system in America would help solve this problem, and that is why I feel a Medicare for All plan would help increase breastfeeding success and rates. Health care should be a *right* rather than just a benefit, and we need to cover every American citizen. It is stupid not to because this results in health and social inequities that cause medical and social problems that cost billions of medical/social care dollars to treat. Health is our greatest wealth, and when we don't protect it by giving everyone the health care they need (especially our vulnerable new mothers and babies!), we all pay with the ill health of our American society.

The likelihood of successful and extended breastfeeding correlates with many factors. Mothers who are better educated, higher income, well-resourced, older, white, and have two-parent families are much more likely to successfully breastfeed and for longer. However, the most vulnerable babies in America are the least likely to be breastfed and are weaned to formula much earlier. This is due to the many barriers their mothers endure: poverty, illness, too early a return to work, work in unsupportive employment, lack of medical insurance and other benefits from employment, single parenthood, lack of support and resources, prematurity, neurocognitive issues, racial inequities, etcetera. Yet it is these most vulnerable babies who are the most negatively affected by the ill effects of formula feeding! Then their lack of being breastfed contributes to their inability to get out of poverty and inequity, and they have increased needs/costs for medical care and social services—coupled with a loss of health insurance coverage for the Medicaid mother at six weeks postpartum. Health care insurance for everyone, including *all* mothers and babies, would help them to receive the needed lactation services they need and deserve and not have to rush back to work just for health insurance coverage.

Breastfeeding for Empowerment and Equity

Breastfeeding success is empowering for a mother and her family, as they don't have to depend on and spend time, money, and resources on a costly but inferior product for their baby! Another way of saying this, which I commonly use in my discussions with mothers-to-be in WIC, is *"Breastfeeding is a resource, while formula feeding is an outsource,"* or *"Breastfeeding is mom-made, while formula feeding is man-made."* In WIC, a mother who is fully breastfeeding receives a much bigger food package for 12 months after the baby's birth, while formula-feeding mothers receive about half as much food for only six months due to the high cost of formula in the WIC package.

Also, WIC never gives enough formula for a baby, so the formula-feeding family is forced to spend more of their own money on extra formula that their baby needs as well as more money spent on medical care. Formula feeding is an extra financial and resource burden for the non-breastfeeding family who is low-income already. This doesn't make sense, but due to the higher breastfeeding barriers that many low-income WIC mothers experience, WIC's free formula ends up being too tempting an enticement. Then, formula supplementation causes babies not to breastfeed as often, decreasing a mother's milk production. This often results in an earlier-than-intended weaning to fully formula feeding. More about the economics of breastfeeding versus formula feeding and WIC follows in the next chapter.

Breastfeeding also enhances an involved and interactive mothering/parenting style that continues long after the child is weaned. This improves family cohesiveness because of the improved bonding that is a benefit of breastfeeding and influenced by breastfeeding hormones, which a formula-feeding mother lacks. This strong mother/baby attachment helps to ameliorate the stresses of single parenting, home and family instability, and lack of resources that some WIC families experience. It is also known to decrease the incidence of neglect or abuse of children.

Summary

When most mothers and babies (of all ethnicities, education, income, origin, genders, sexual identities, ages, and other diversities) can enjoy equitable breastfeeding support and benefits, we will all enjoy greater equity, better health, and deeper understanding through our experience of breastfeeding our babies! The common denominator of successful breastfeeding is that it ameliorates and transcends the many differences and inequities in America. As Americans, we mothers would benefit by having this breastfeeding experience in common and in *equity* in our "melting pot of the world." We are all stakeholders in the support and the benefits gained from breastfeeding! The societal benefits and economic savings resulting from breastfeeding could more than cover paid family leave if mothers were able to breastfeed more exclusively and for longer. A national paid family leave and comprehensive health care coverage for all in America would help reduce the need for breastfeeding mothers to return to work before breastfeeding is well established and cover the needed lactation services they deserve to help them do the important work of breastfeeding their babies.

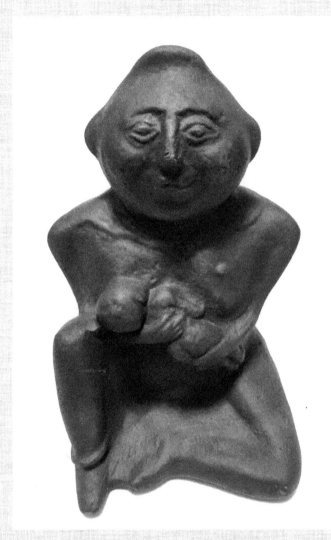

The Mississippian culture commemorated breastfeeding with sculptures like this replica of a nursing mother figurine, dated about BC 1300, found at Cahokia Mounds, a city that was once home to as many as 40,000 Native Americans during its peak in the 12th century AD due to its central location along trade routes.

— 4 —

Economic Health

Breastfeeding saves money for families, health care systems, and societies. Breastfeeding is a self-produced and on-demand system that saves families a lot of money, resources, time, and effort when it is going well. Breastfeeding mothers do not need to buy an expensive product and go to all the effort that purchasing and preparing an externally produced, for-profit product entails. One-time costs involved in breastfeeding include breastfeeding-related products like a breastfeeding bra and a Boppy pillow, some bottles if a mother works, a pump if not free from the insurance company, or an appointment with a lactation professional, but they are minimal compared to the costs of formula. Breastfeeding's true costs are in the time and work a mother spends doing it, which is completely ignored in the US.

Not breastfeeding costs money and adds financial burden to the most vulnerable while lining the pockets of corporations. Infant formula use ranges from 15 to 40 ounces per day, and formula costs range from approximately $1,000 to $3,000 per year without considering the additional costs of equipment and extra medical costs. Babies are more likely to overfeed from bottles, as they don't have to work at the feed like they do with direct breastfeeding. Overfeeding at any age causes lots of acute and chronic health problems and wastes money and resources. The costs of formula, water, bottles, nipples, cleaning supplies, extra doctor visits, medicine, and time off work to tend to the baby with more illnesses add up for individual families. These costs are extra burdens to families who are already burdened with the increased barriers to breastfeeding present due to poverty, lack of education and resources, no paid family leave, and marginal employment.

The people who qualify for WIC are the same people who qualify for Medicaid. Medicaid spends more health care dollars on children who are formula fed than on those who are breastfed. Each child who isn't breastfed adds to our Medicaid costs, since formula-fed infants are sick more often and more seriously. The consequences of not breastfeeding also show up as chronic illness later in life for both mom and baby, causing suffering, disability, and greater medical care expenditures. In America, chronic illness medical care eats up a huge portion of our health care dollars and is much costlier than childhood illnesses, yet we haven't done a comprehensive analysis of how many medical care dollars could be saved if mothers and babies breastfed for longer in America. A system that lacks breastfeeding recognition and support and serves up formula feeding on a silver platter is robbing a mother of her self-production capacity and forcing her to buy into the formula and medical industries.

WIC and Formula Subsidies

Although formula is an inferior form of infant nutrition compared to breast milk/breastfeeding, our government subsidizes the formula industry through WIC. WIC started giving vouchers for formula in the late 1970s and now provides *more than half of the formula that is used in the US*. WIC breastfeeding rates are much lower than the national average for both initiation and continuation breastfeeding rates because WIC mothers return to work sooner due to financial necessity, and they return to workplaces that are less supportive of breastfeeding. WIC provides breastfeeding education and support as required by law, but the free formula entices many mothers to succumb to its use when they return to work early or have breastfeeding problems. WIC gives breastfeeding support by hiring lactation professionals and peer counselors to promote, educate, and support breastfeeding mothers and babies; it also makes pumps available to breastfeeding moms as needed and does outreach in communities to promote/support breastfeeding, but the funding for this pales in relation to the WIC funds spent on formula subsidies.

To save money on formula costs, WIC instituted a competitive bidding process that generally yields $1 to $2 billion a year in rebates. Subsequently, WIC pays on average only 5% to 15% of the formula's wholesale cost, but formula cost is still a substantial amount of the total WIC budget. For example, in 2010, the total WIC budget was around $7 billion with WIC formula costs being close to $1 billion. In 2013, approximately $1.88 billion in rebates were received for food-related costs, mostly from infant formula rebates. That year, a total of $6.38 billion was spent on WIC, with $1.88 billion offset by rebates (mostly for formula), which reduced from 30% to around 23% the total proportion of food costs, of which the greatest amount of dollars goes to formula.

Comparatively, the cost of all nutrition education, including a much smaller portion of the nutrition education specifically for breastfeeding promotion and support, was only $559 million in 2013. Nationally, about 34% of Nutrition Services and Administration (NSA) grant funds were spent on program management, 37% was spent on client services, 21% was spent on nutrition education, and only 8% on breastfeeding support. Breastfeeding support obviously gets the short end of WIC funding.

WIC serves around 1.8 to 2 million infants born in the US per year (which is around 50%). Due to a shrinking market for formula, because of higher breastfeeding rates among the non-WIC mothers, formula manufacturers compete aggressively for WIC contracts to maintain their sales. This heavy WIC formula funding means that the formula industry is being subsidized by our government even though it entails the use of an inferior product for our most vulnerable babies. WIC's huge subsidies for formula (and too little subsidy of breastfeeding) is not a good recipe for encouraging breastfeeding among WIC participants. Mothers and babies inflicted with poverty (and all the issues that tag along with poverty) are much more likely to suffer from the ills of not breastfeeding that cause a continuation of their impoverished status.

WIC's breastfeeding rates are going up slowly but are substantially less than the breastfeeding rates of non-WIC mothers. The question is, does WIC's free formula dilute WIC's breastfeeding support efforts? It is hard not to surmise that the substantial WIC subsidy of formula is a product endorsement that lessens a mother's incentive to breastfeed, or breastfeed for as long, resulting in lower WIC breastfeeding rates. If the WIC subsidy amounts were gradually redirected away from so much formula and toward more breastfeeding support and improved breastfeeding food packages, it is likely that we would reduce health care spending while giving greater incentive for WIC mothers to breastfeed. This should be done gradually so that we can reduce the current overreliance on formula, while as a nation, we commit to making breastfeeding easier for our mothers and children by following the recommendations in this book. (Taking away formula subsidies WITHOUT giving additional breastfeeding and nutritional support is NOT what I am talking about!)

Extra funding for breastfeeding support in WIC could include enhanced and extended breastfeeding food packages for breastfeeding moms who breastfeed for longer than one year, more breastfeeding support staff hired and placed in all WIC centers (some WIC centers do not currently have breastfeeding support), and more breastfeeding supplies for breastfeeding mothers. Currently, WIC ends food packages for the breastfeeding mom at one year regardless of whether she is still breastfeeding. An improved and extended food package for the breastfeeding mom might serve as a good incentive for mothers to breastfeed for longer and might allow for mothers to reduce their work hours with a better food package and reduced food costs.

Breastfeeding doesn't mean a baby will never get ill. All babies get ill as part of the development of their immune systems, but fully breastfed (exclusively breastfed for six months and continued breastfeeding until one year or more) babies are sick less often and less seriously and have reduced risks of chronic illness later in life. This saves a lot of anxiety, suffering, and lost sleep for parents and money spent on medical care. Wouldn't we, as a nation, want to do everything possible to reduce human suffering and, at the same time, minimize these economic costs, especially for the most vulnerable in our society—our young babies and families?

Paying More for an Inferior Product: Formula

Go to the store and look at the current formula ingredient lists, and you'll see the first and foremost ingredient is often corn syrup, which indicates it is the principal ingredient—even before the milk ingredient! Most corn syrup is genetically modified and certainly is a poor nutritional substitute for the healthy milk-based carbohydrates in breast milk.

Below are formula ingredients, copied off labels at the grocery store. Note that the main ingredients are listed in order of the amount used, so the first ingredient is the largest amount:

Formula #1: **Corn syrup solids (54%),** vegetable oil (26%), protein isolate (14%)...

Formula #2: **Corn syrup solids (48%),** vegetable oils (26%), casein hydrolysate milk (17%), modified corn starch (4%)...

Formula #3: **Corn syrup solids (39%),** soy protein isolate (14%), high oleic safflower oil (11%), **sugar (10%),** soy oil (8%), coconut oil (8%)...

Many don't list the percentages of ingredients, but the fact that corn syrup is the first listed ingredient means it the largest amount:

Formula #4: **Corn syrup**, milk protein isolate, high oleic safflower oil, **sugar**, soy oil, coconut oil, galacto-oligosaccharides...

Formula #5: **Corn syrup**, nonfat milk, palm olein, whey protein hydrolysate, coconut oil, soy oil, high oleic safflower or sunflower oil...

Formula #6: **Corn syrup solids**, partially hydrolyzed nonfat milk and whey protein concentrate solids (soy), vegetable oil (palm olein, soy and coconut and high oleic and sunflower oils)...

Formula #7: **Corn syrup solids,** vegetable oil, partially hydrogenated nonfat milk, whey protein...

Formula #8: **Corn maltodextrin**, whey protein concentrate, vegetable oils...

Some don't have corn syrup as the first ingredient:

Formula #9: Partially hydrolyzed nonfat (cow's) milk, whey protein concentrate, vegetable oil, **corn syrup solids,** lactose…

Formula #10: Nonfat (cow's) milk, **lactose**, vegetable oils, whey protein concentrate… (This one has lactose instead of corn syrup.)

The rest of the ingredients of each type of formula compose "less than 2%" of the total ingredients and include various added vitamins, but I am not listing them here.

Human milk's principal carbohydrate is lactose, as noted in Olivia Ballard and Ardythe L. Morrow's analysis "Human Milk Composition: Nutrients and Bioactive Factors," published in the medical journal *Pediatric Clinics of North America* in 2014:

"The principal sugar of human milk is the disaccharide lactose. The concentration of lactose in human milk is the least variable of the macronutrients…. The other significant carbohydrates of human milk are the oligosaccharides, which comprise approximately 1 g/dL in human milk, depending on stage of lactation and maternal genetic factors."

Corn syrup as a carbohydrate is very different than the natural milk sugars of breast milk. Corn syrup causes a higher glycemic index and more work for the baby's pancreas, which can predispose a baby to higher risk of obesity and diabetes. It is also genetically modified, which brings up other concerns. Do we really want to be feeding this to our babies in their first year of life—when they're growing the fastest and in their most vulnerable year of life?

The Economic Value of Breastfeeding

The monetary costs of formula are small compared to the costs mothers and families incur from not breastfeeding and the costs babies pay from not being breastfed. A thorough economic analysis has not been done on this important public health issue due to our country's tendency to ignore women's issues in favor of man-made products that involve money, resources, and profit. In other words, our country's failure to place a value on breastfeeding is indicative of our sexist and capitalistic tendencies in America.

We need a national analysis of the economic benefits of breastfeeding and the real costs of not breastfeeding, as has been done with the costs of environmental degradation, smoking, or not wearing seatbelts or helmets in America. This economic analysis should include the upfront costs of formula and supplies, government-subsidized WIC formula costs, the higher medical costs of formula-fed infants, and the costs of lost productivity due to increased morbidity and mortality from lack of breastfeeding. This economic analysis should cover both the child and mother's health status as both are affected by breastfeeding or not breastfeeding. After this economic analysis is completed, then including breastfeeding (the active and involved delivery of breast milk) as a part of our gross national product (GNP) would help us to recognize and value its part in our economic system and would give the recognition and support breastfeeding mothers deserve. Then this analysis could be used as a rationale for paid family leave in America.

In her 2014 conference paper "'Lost Milk?' – The Economic Value of Breastmilk in GDP," health researcher Julie P. Smith says:

The value of human milk can be measured using accepted international guidelines for calculating national income and production. The market value of this commodity is quantitatively nontrivial and should be counted in GDP based on UN national accounting guidelines. Not accounting for mothers' milk production in GDP and other economic data biases public policy. The invisibility of human milk reduces the perceived importance of programs and regulations that protect and support women to breastfeed. The potential lost of economic production from not protecting women's lactation and milk production from competing pressures such as employment and commercial marketing is large.

An Economic Study of Breastfeeding and Impact on Medical Spending

In 2018, Americans spent approximately $3.6 trillion on health/medical care costs, which is greater than $11,000 per person per year. That is much more than any other health care system in the world. Yet we aren't enjoying the best health compared to many other countries, as evidenced by having higher infant mortality rates, lower longevity rates, and many costly chronic health problems. It is frustrating, especially to those of us who know the many benefits of breastfeeding, that we do only small, limited studies in the US on how breastfeeding saves a few billion health care dollars. It is also frustrating to see so much health care funding (83%) go to tertiary (highly specialized medical care to treat chronic illnesses) medical care and less than 5% go to primary (wellness) health care, like breastfeeding support. The rest goes to secondary care (early treatment of an illness) costs. America has a bad, bad habit of succumbing to the sensational and profiteering methods of tertiary (illness) care and ignoring the primary (wellness) care funding. Then, because we do not invest in primary care, our tertiary care needs, costs, and poor outcomes are much higher! Breastfeeding is a potent form of primary health care for both mother and baby and deserves more recognition and funding!

Using just one illness that is higher due to non-breastfeeding—diabetes—as an example on how many health/medical care dollars could be saved if breastfeeding rates were increased gives a good perspective. In 2017, diabetes cost $237 billion in medical care expenditures and $90 billion in reduced productivity costs. This accounts for approximately one out of every 10 dollars spent on health care in America! Diabetes is now considered an epidemic in America, with one out of eight Americans having diabetes, many more with prediabetes, and predictions of much higher rates and costs of diabetes in the future! Some are predicting that one out of every three to five Americans will have diabetes in our near future. The problem of diabetes is referred to as the elephant in the room that is not being heeded (enough) even as it is trampling on our quality of life and economic and health care systems.

A good dose of breastfeeding significantly reduces the (later) incidence of diabetes for the baby *and* mother (around 40% reduction for two people—mother and baby). I discussed how breastfeeding reduces diabetes, obesity, and metabolic disease, which usually go hand in hand, in the first chapter. If we can increase breastfeeding rates to our national goals, we could eventually reduce our spending for diabetes significantly (using the 40% reduction in diabetes incidence from breastfeeding for a year) for mother and baby, *saving many billions of dollars* on that one illness alone! It would take some time to see these health changes and health care dollar savings because we must undo several generations of non-breastfeeding epigenetics, but if we don't start soon, we will be furthering our reliance on expensive and painful tertiary care illness and the expenditures for diabetes and other chronic illnesses associated with not breastfeeding.

I have included CDC maps in Chapter 7 showing how the incidence of lower breastfeeding rates are correlated with higher obesity and diabetes rates in America. One graph shows that the rate of diabetes started rising when the breastfeeding rates were lowest in America. The diabetes rate increases are seen to be slowing slightly in the most recent years. This could be related to the slowly rising rates of breastfeeding initiation over the past 50 years in America. Imagine what improved breastfeeding *continuation* rates, with better breastfeeding support in America, might do in stemming the rise of diabetes, obesity, and associated metabolic disease incidence!

We know that breastfeeding reduces the incidence of many more illnesses for both the mother and baby in terms of both acute and chronic illnesses, so many more health care dollars could be saved and reallocated to primary health care and paid family leave! Some of our most common and expensive illnesses such as breast cancer, heart disease, obesity, and metabolic disease could be reduced substantially by greater breastfeeding success and rates for both mother and baby! *What other public health practice is so effective?!* It is frustrating that so little economic research into breastfeeding has been done in the US! There are a few, but they use the reduction in the short-term (acute) illnesses to study breastfeeding as it relates to medical dollars saved and come up with a few billion dollars saved. We need to study how breastfeeding reduces chronic illnesses to really see how breastfeeding saves dollars! Then we would see how effective breastfeeding is as a public health issue with savings in hundreds of billions of dollars.

Summary

This chapter on the economic issues of breastfeeding versus formula feeding shows just how much money is being wasted on formula, an inferior product. Yet the inclusion of breastfeeding as a cost-saving health tool is ignored. A comprehensive economic cost/benefit analysis of breastfeeding, based on accurate breastfeeding data collected and documented on every baby, is doable and needed. It starts with accurate and comprehensive breastfeeding data on every baby, which I discussed in the first chapter. If we start by assessing comprehensive breastfeeding statistics and documenting them on health care charts, it will be apparent how effective breastfeeding is in reducing illness and saving dollars. It begins with "counting" breastfeeding and doing an economic study of the issue of breastfeeding in our society and health/medical care system. That which gets comprehensively counted and documented gets the attention, funding, and analysis it needs to be put to good use, as well as the ability to see how effective that issue is related to health care dollars saved.

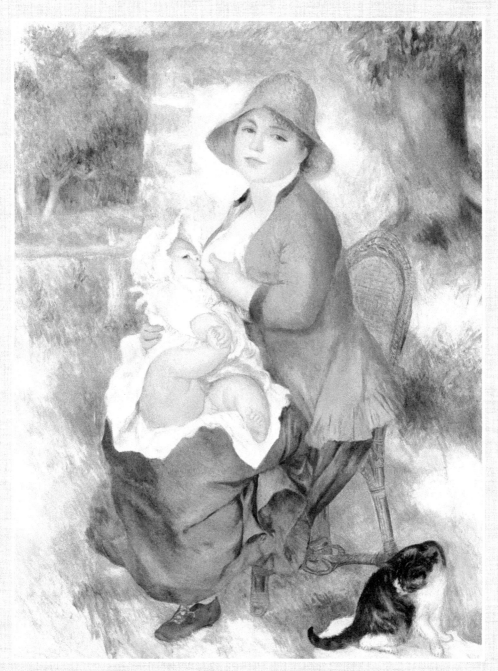

Motherhood (aka *Woman Breast Feeding Her Child*), by Pierre-Auguste Renoir, 1886.

— 5 —

Environmental Health

Breastfeeding is environmentally friendly and decreases pollution. Here are some of the ways breastfeeding is "green" compared to formula:

- Breastfeeding creates no pollution or production emissions and contributes a lot less "packaging" (aluminum cans, plastic bottles, nipples, paper, and cleaning supplies) and other waste to our landfills.
- Breastfeeding does not use water, fuel, electricity, storage space, and utilities for production, transport, and refrigeration in homes, stores, or hospitals.
- Breastfeeding is fresh and natural and uses no genetically modified (GMO) ingredients such as corn syrup—the first ingredient in many formulas—and soy products in soy-based formulas.
- Breast milk contains less chemicals, pesticides, and antibiotics than formula.
- Breastfeeding results in less pasture land usage for cows, less water usage for cows, less cow feed, less antibiotics in cow feed, less cow dung, and less methane gas.
- Breastfeeding reduces hospitalizations of babies and lessens the use of medicines, medical equipment, and toxic medical waste.
- Breastfeeding mothers have a slower birth rate and use less menstrual products due to <u>lactational amenorrhea</u>.

Breastfeeding has a positive impact on our environment and our health. On the other hand, the formula industry increases the pollution of our environment—and receives government subsidies even while it does so! Just look at all the ways that breastfeeding protects the environment versus the flip side: how much formula feeding pollutes our environment. The use (and pollution) of our land, water, and resources due to production and use of cow milk–based formula (most of formula is made from cow's milk) is a huge detriment to our environment. The heavy use of antibiotics in animal feed is a form of pollution. The greatest use of antibiotics is for animal feed and is the main cause of antibiotic resistance. The heavy use of pesticides in growing the corn for animal feed is pollution. The worsened health status of our mothers and babies and the greater need for medical care is another form of pollution stemming from formula usage. The funding subsidies for formula is a monetized type of pollution that sequesters funding and causes too little to be left over for the support of breastfeeding.

The dairy industry receives a lot of subsidies from our government. WIC started in the 1970s, when dairy farmers had too much product for too little demand, so the government created the WIC program to help both the farmers and those women and children in poverty. This is one strong reason why WIC is so heavily influenced by the dairy industry and demonstrates yet another way in which national policies and services have been influenced by corporate industries in America. So, the US government spends WIC dollars to subsidize formula feeding, which benefits dairy farmers and the pharmaceutical companies that sell the formula, as well as the babies who need formula, even though they are getting an inferior product.

Heavy reliance and subsidies for formula add up to pollution not only at the environmental level, but also pollution of government services supporting the use of an inferior product. That, in turn, results in a lot of waste, pollution, and expenditures in our health care system. Wouldn't it make sense to reduce breastfeeding barriers, increase breastfeeding support, reduce WIC formula expenditures gradually and reapply them to support breastfeeding, fund more milk banks, and legislate a national paid family leave so that mothers could be more successful with breastfeeding? Our physical and social environments would benefit as well!

Breastfeeding as a Recognized, Valued, and Protected Natural Resource

Breastfeeding is a biological necessity for the health and well-being of mothers and infants. It is a natural resource! When other natural resources have been seen as essential to the health and well-being of the population, legislative recognition, protection, and funding for those natural resources have been put in place. One example is green spaces and all the national and state parks in the US. There are theories and methods for determining the value of natural resources. Once a natural resource is given a value within our social and economic systems, it can be given protection. What if breastfeeding, or breast milk, was considered a natural resource and given a value in our systems? If it can be done with other natural resources, it can be done with breastfeeding/breast milk and will lead to protections and supports for this potent natural resource. Many books, articles, and classes discuss how to value and protect other natural resources, and we can follow those same guidelines for breastfeeding as a natural resource.

Breastfeeding could then be given a status as a <u>gross domestic product (GDP)</u>, which would help our country to establish and fund a national paid leave system in that it would support breastfeeding as a natural resource worth protection. It would also enable other supports, such as funding for more lactation consultants, more breastfeeding education programs for other health care professionals, and more laws, policies, and research that support breastfeeding. Just like the Environmental Protection Agency (EPA) was created in 1970 for the purpose of environmental protection, a Breastfeeding Protection Agency could be established to protect breastfeeding as the natural resource it is!

Giving a value and status for breastfeeding as a natural resource, as has been done with natural resources by environmental economists, will help America to recognize the worth of breastfeeding. Making breastfeeding a part of our GDP, based on the assessment of its value in reducing health and social costs, will give it this status and recognizable worth. When we have accurately assessed, counted, and assigned a value to breastfeeding as a natural resource and potent public health tool, we will have convincing data to enact breastfeeding support and protection measures. Breastfeeding can then be utilized as a potent tool for health, economic, social, and environmental equity in the US.

Human Milk Banks

Brazil is a county committed to reducing their high infant mortality rate by increasing breastfeeding and human milk feeding. Brazil now has 213 milk banks; the US has only 25 milk banks. Why doesn't the US have more human milk banks?

In the US, there are over 800 neonatal intensive care units (NICUs), where premature and very sick babies are cared for by specialists. Many neonatologist MDs want human milk for their patients when their mothers are unable to provide their own milk. In 2017, over five million ounces of banked human milk were distributed, but these fragile babies usually only received banked milk for a few weeks. More milk banks are needed to serve the needs of these NICU babies who are at greater risk for serious illnesses due to their fragility. Banked milk is also being requested for older babies and adults who have illnesses, but that is rarely accomplished due to the lack of banked milk available. Having more milk banks would decrease our reliance on formula when moms are not able to or choose not to breastfeed and would help to ensure human milk for human babies instead of artificial, man-made formulas. There are thousands of blood banks in the US, and although there is less need for human milk than blood, we definitely need more milk banks than the current 25 in the US. Almost 3.8 million babies were born in the US in 2018, and although we don't know what percentage of babies will need banked milk, we should at least have a human milk bank associated with each pediatric NICU hospital in the US.

See the Notes section at the end of this book for resources on milk banks.

Breastfeeding and Human Milk Research

In the 2016 TED talk by Katie Hinde on "What We Don't Know About Mother's Milk," she points out that there is more research at the National Institutes of Health on coffee, wine, and tomatoes than there is on human milk. Of the National Institutes of Health's holdings of approximately 25 million research articles, there are less than 100,000 on lactation or breast milk, and there is more than twice as much research on erectile dysfunction than on breastfeeding and human milk. A huge amount of research on cow's milk exists, but so much less on human milk, which is the first and foremost nourishment for our young and vulnerable babies.

Why is funding for breastfeeding research so hard to come by yet research funds for other issues and substances are abundant? I think it is because breastfeeding is not a moneymaker and doesn't reap profit for a company or business, and our profit-motivated system does not allocate adequate funding for this reason. Yet, breastfeeding is a money-saver for the breastfeeding mothers, babies, and families as well as our health care system at large, so it deserves ample funding for needed research!

We need more research about breastfeeding and human milk in so many areas of this comprehensive issue: the anatomy and physiology of breastfeeding and breast milk production; the nutritional, hormonal, and immunological science of human milk; the health benefits of breastfeeding as it relates to exclusive versus partial breastfeeding and the duration of breastfeeding for mother and infant; the medical issues that impact breastfeeding; how the birth style impacts breastfeeding initiation and success; the social issues affecting breastfeeding experience; the barriers to breastfeeding and how best to reduce them; the most effective methods and tools for breastfeeding support; medications and their impacts on breast milk production, milk quality, and the infant; how foods and nutrition affect the breastfeeding mother and her milk production; environmental toxins and their effect on human milk; human milk banking and safe human milk sharing; pumps and other breastfeeding products; lactational amenorrhea and birth spacing; metabolic disease, including obesity, and its impact on breastfeeding and how much breastfeeding reduces metabolic disease; best methods to enhance milk production for mothers with insufficient milk supply; the epigenetic changes associated with many generations of non-breastfeeding; how laws, policies, medical, social, and cultural issues impact breastfeeding; and the economics of breastfeeding, as I mentioned before.

As Katie Hinde said in her TED talk, "that we know so much less about breast milk, the first fluid a young mammal is adapted to consume, should make us angry." The lack of research and funding for research on breastfeeding and human milk is stunting our ability as a nation to be successful with promoting and supporting our breastfeeding mothers and babies.

Summary
This chapter illuminates the environmental benefits of breastfeeding. The environmental consequences and costs related to non-breastfeeding include the pollution of the natural environment as well as within our social and political realms. Protecting and supporting breastfeeding and human milk as the natural resource it is would be so much healthier for our environment, our health, and our society. More research into the worthy subject of breastfeeding and human milk is needed, and so is more funding for human milk banks in all major cities.

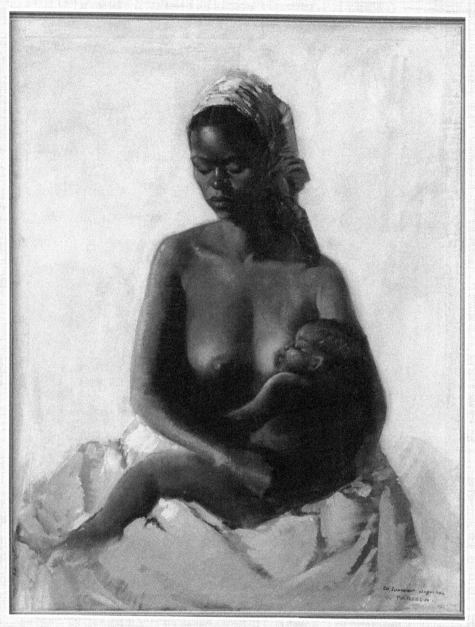

Gaston Parison (1889–1959) was a French artist who depicted scenes of mothers breast-feeding their babies during his time in Africa. This photo of *African Mother and Child* is printed courtesy of Galerie St-John, Ghent, Belgium.

— 6 —

Maternal Empowerment

Maternal empowerment is an important benefit of breastfeeding that often goes unrecognized. In 1956, the founders of La Leche League—seven mothers in Illinois who started what they thought would be a local, temporary breastfeeding support group—were quite savvy about the importance of empowering mothers through breastfeeding. They called it "Mothering through Breastfeeding." It is the same principle as the old saying, "give a man a fish and you feed him for a day; teach a man to fish and you feed him for a lifetime." Supporting mothers to breastfeed empowers them by allowing them to self-produce the best nutrition for their babies and not be forced to rely on the inferior products of formula and the ensuing need for more tertiary medical care.

Teaching, promoting, and supporting mothers to breastfeed their babies empowers them in the following ways:

1. Protects and enhances the mothering role.
2. Self-production of breast milk: no need to buy expensive formula.
3. Keeps mom and baby healthier and less dependent on medical care system.
4. More control over the feeding process: process oriented rather than product oriented.
5. Improved bonding and knowing about one's baby. Knowledge is power.
6. Maternal confidence builder: seeing baby thrive on her own milk!
7. Enhanced mothering skills and a great comforting tool for babies.
8. Saves money, resources, and time when breastfeeding is going well.
9. Self-control: using your own breasts for your and baby's needs/desires.
10. Feminism at its best: empowers mothering through self-production.

In my opinion, empowering mothers and babies is one of the most precious benefits of breastfeeding. When a mother receives the support she needs and deserves to be successful with breastfeeding, she is empowered to provide the best for herself and her baby and is less reliant on others or costly products or medical care services. Everyone benefits when mothers are supported and empowered to breastfeed!

La Leche League Founders Deserve a Nobel Peace Prize

The founders of La Leche League (LLL) deserve recognition for their enduring contributions to all the mothers and babies they have helped through their mother-to-mother volunteer breastfeeding support organization for over 63 years! LLL is now represented in over 65 countries and is recognized as the world authority on breastfeeding. LLL has been the main reason that the "womanly art of breastfeeding" has not been lost in most developed countries.

It is important that the Founders of La Leche League and the organization be recognized for the invaluable contribution to the health and well-being of our world at large through supporting and furthering the womanly art of breastfeeding. I would think the Founders would have been awarded a Nobel Peace Prize and/or other recognition that they so richly deserve for their many years of volunteer work supporting breastfeeding! What is more peaceful than a healthy baby receiving the best nutrition and immune protection, sensory enrichment, and nurturance at their *empowered* mother's breast? Also, since LLL work is all volunteer-based, that makes it even more deserving of awards! So why have the La Leche League Founders not been awarded a Nobel Peace Prize or a Presidential Medal or other significant awards?! Too few women are recognized and awarded the Nobel Prize and other awards, and this would be a chance to help correct that huge discrepancy! Women have only been the recipients of fewer than 6% of Nobel Prizes, yet women are over 50% of the population! This is yet another example of how women and women's issues are ignored by our patriarchal society.

Breastfeeding: The Womanly Art

Breastfeeding art historically was prolific, but it decreased in America around the same time that breastfeeding rates decreased. For an example, religious art used to commonly depict Mother Mary breastfeeding Jesus. Historical breastfeeding art showed that a woman's ability to breastfeed was revered and respected and was thought to be a great source of a woman's power! But that all went away, and in America, one rarely sees breastfeeding art now. In America, the bottle became the norm pictured in ads, books, TV, and art. Now that breastfeeding practices are coming back, so should breastfeeding art, since art is life's depiction and a form of recognition and celebration.

Breastfeeding mothers nowadays are taking "brelfies"—selfies of breastfeeding mothers and babies—and mothers are sitting for professional photographs showing them breastfeeding. I encourage all breastfeeding mothers to take photos or have artwork made of yourselves while breastfeeding so you have a visual documentation of your gift to your child and to society. I also invite artists to restart the artistic documentation of breastfeeding in our culture, documenting this important act of nurturance by our mothers!

I would also love to see museums and other public spaces hosting breastfeeding art from historical and current times. It would also be nice to see other art forms documenting breastfeeding through music, theatre, sculpture, and comedy. When the artistic representation of breastfeeding abounds, we will know breastfeeding has returned to America's bosom! A few of my favorite breastfeeding art works from various sources follow or are placed throughout this book.

Breastfeeding Stamps

Another example of our country's tendency to ignore women's issues and deny recognition to forms of women's empowerment is the example of our lack of a breastfeeding postage stamp in America. Many other countries have a breastfeeding stamp as part of their social and governmental recognition, promotion, and support of breastfeeding. Since 1999, some breastfeeding advocates in America have been requesting an American breastfeeding stamp to promote and recognize this important aspect of healthy infant feeding in the US in accordance with our national goals to increase breastfeeding rates and duration. The US Citizens' Stamp Advisory Committee, which reviews all requests for new stamps in America, has said no to all our requests and petitions for many years. We collected many signatures and sent several petitions requesting a breastfeeding stamp in America. There have been many frivolous stamps issued in the meantime, such as the muscle car stamp and other stamps related to cartoons.

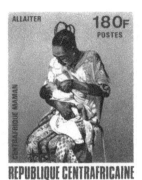

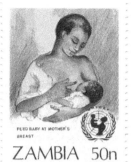

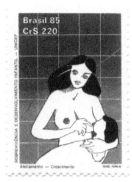

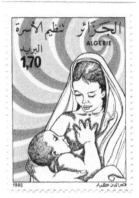

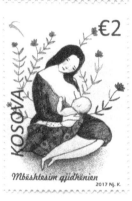

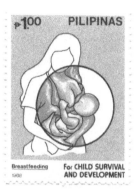

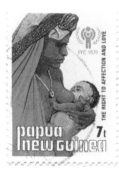

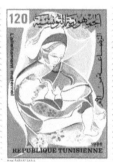

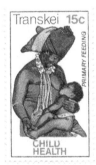

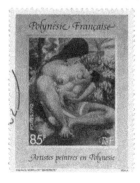

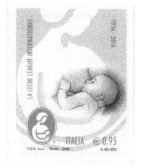

On the other hand, the breast cancer stamp has flourished and has raised millions of dollars for breast cancer support and research! This is an example of our tendency to prioritize tertiary, monetized care over primary care in America. We know that breastfeeding decreases the incidence of breast cancer, so why do we not have a breastfeeding stamp to help decrease the incidence of breast cancer? It is also probably due to "genderized" support for saving the breasts from a male perspective rather than a female perspective. In other words, breast cancer funding, in part, saves breasts for their use filling out a feminine figure, and that might be why a breast cancer stamp has been approved, while a breastfeeding stamp, which promotes breastfeeding for mothers' and babies' benefit, has been denied in the US. Here are just a few photos of breastfeeding stamps from other countries around the world, showing that other countries recognize the importance of depicting breastfeeding as an important aspect of mothering and a potent public health issue. Links to the process of requesting a stamp design from the Citizens' Stamp Advisory Committee are in the Notes section at the end of this book.

Summary

Maternal empowerment is my favorite benefit of breastfeeding, yet it is most often unrecognized. If breastfeeding were recognized as the important act of nurture and empowerment it is, the La Leche League Founders would have been awarded the Nobel, we would have more breastfeeding art in our museums and other social institutions, there would be a USPS breastfeeding stamp, and many other manners of recognition in our society and nation!

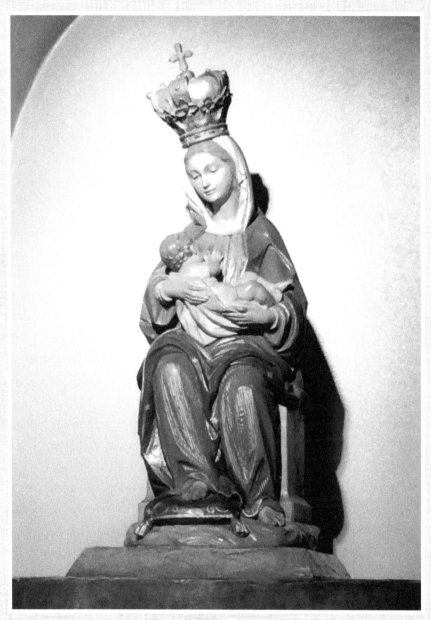

Nuestra Señora de Leche y Buen Parto (Our Lady of Milk and Good Birth). This statue, circa AD 1600–1620, is kept in the shrine devoted to Nuestra Señora de Leche y Buen Parto in St. Augustine, Florida—the first Marian shrine in the United States. The founders of La Leche League took inspiration from Nuestra Señora when naming the organization in 1956, when "breastfeeding" was a risqué word. Photo by Humberto Quintanilla.

—7—

Social Health

The well-being of our family, educational, business, and social institutions also benefit from breastfeeding. When babies are healthier, in all the ways breastfeeding promotes health, it has a positive effect on the whole family and all of society.

Breastfed babies not only have better physical health, but also enjoy improved mental and developmental health due to the intensive bonding and well-being they experience at their mother's breast. They spend more time in mother's arms receiving more sensory-rich and pleasurable stimulation, which improves brain and sensory development. Their eyes, their jaws and teeth, and their kinesthetic sense are all better developed—all due to the biomechanical process of breastfeeding. They are able to devote more energy to growth, development, and learning since they expend less energy combating illness. These are benefits in addition to the unique, bioactive, dynamic, and more bioavailable nutrients of breastfeeding. Breast milk also contains stem cells that migrate from the gut to the brain. (Yes, we breastfeeding mamas do get into our children's brains and have lifelong influence!) These are just some of the reasons for the improved intelligence of breastfed babies. A number of studies have statistically quantified this improved intelligence. Breastfed babies who receive a good dose of breastfeeding (not just token breastfeeding for a short time) have higher IQs when tested later, even when poverty, inequities, or other social disadvantages are present.

This enhanced nurturing and developmental relationship that occurs with successful breastfeeding helps to protect babies against poverty and social inequities. This is because breastfeeding tends to "suck" mothers into their mothering role (to use a play on words). There is too little research about breastfeeding in general, and a paucity of research on the benefits of breastfeeding with regards to the mothering role. However, if there was more research, I know a positive effect on mothering would be noted. It probably also would be noted that there is a positive effect on family cohesiveness as well. It could be that fathers/partners are also "sucked" into the role of supporting this intensive mother/baby relationship that breastfeeding naturally encourages, and this support might be the reason that breastfeeding families might experience greater cohesiveness. What is well known and documented is that breastfeeding leads to less child neglect, abandonment, and abuse!

From a personal perspective: My son went to public school, where he qualified for the gifted school program. In my discussions with other mothers at school functions, we often discussed how we fed our babies, and many had breastfed. We had a strong parent–teacher organization and a lot of parental involvement in the school and extracurricular activities. My guess is that the percentage of children in the gifted program who were breastfed was higher. I do know that parental involvement in the gifted program was much higher than in other public schools. The early investment and intimacy of breastfeeding tends to draw mothers and supportive fathers into being strongly vested in their child's development. This attachment endures long after breastfeeding has ended! This often leads to continued involvement in their children's education long term. It is well recognized that the more parents are involved in a child's education, the better that child does in school. The improved physical, developmental, and intellectual health of breastfed babies and the more involved parenting translate into fewer behavioral and cognitive issues in school and less time away from school due to illness or behavioral problems. This leads to a better education, and a better education leads to a better job and higher income, which can significantly improve quality of life and functioning within society.

Although prison inmates suffer from many social ills, many who land in prison have had a history of problems in school and behavioral and/or mental health problems. It would be interesting to know if people who end up in prisons were breastfed and for how long, but we do not have the comprehensive breastfeeding statistics we need to know this. Not being breastfed doesn't mean a person is more likely to commit a crime, but I do believe that the same barriers causing babies not to be breastfed are the same reasons some babies might land in prison when they are grown. Breastfeeding *and the nurturance that comes in tandem* with breastfeeding serve as primary health tools to ameliorate and even prevent some social ills that often come with poverty. We need to reduce barriers and give better support so that all babies from all backgrounds can be breastfed, with the best and most unique *nutrition and nurturance* to meet their unique needs for the healthiest growth and development.

Since there is much too little breastfeeding research in the US, we don't have all these social benefits well documented, but they are recognized by many, and we need to research these social benefits! A good population to study for these social and family benefits of breastfeeding would be a population of La Leche League mothers and their babies, as they tend to breastfeed more exclusively and for longer due to getting support from La Leche League. It might be argued that mothers who seek La Leche League support have characteristics that are associated with longer and more successful breastfeeding habits, and this would have to be controlled for, but this would be a good group to study for breastfeeding research. Also, WIC breastfeeding mothers could be a good resource for breastfeeding research. The mothering and parental/social benefits of breastfeeding need and deserve to be studied, as this improved family health and cohesiveness is a huge benefit to society!

I've pointed out many reasons that breastfeeding mothers, babies, and families are healthier and socially hardier: moms experience health benefits from breastfeeding empowerment and convenience; babies are healthier and smarter from the better nutrition, immunity, and the enriched sensory stimulation of breastfeeding; they tend to do better in school, having fewer missed school days for illness; they enjoy enhanced neurocognitive development; families enjoy a greater likelihood for parental involvement, which persists long after breastfeeding ends; and families save a lot of money! This healthier childhood and greater time and involvement in school lead to improved chances of success in a breastfed baby's adult life! A healthier baby grows up to be a healthier citizen of our shared world!

These educational and social benefits of breastfeeding go way beyond the nutritional and immune benefits, and they last a lifetime, making life easier for those that received the "special recipe" and nurturance that comes from a mother through breastfeeding! Mothers also gain health and social benefits from breastfeeding by improved health, convenience, monetary savings, and the satisfaction/confidence she gains from breastfeeding, which results in less reliance on others (formula industry/medical system) for her and her baby's well-being. This work of breastfeeding, which has many social benefits, needs support from all institutions who gain from a breastfed baby who grows up to become a healthy, hardy adult: educational, economic, employment, environmental, community, health care, business, and government systems! Next, I am going to discuss how employers need to support breastfeeding.

Breastfeeding Support in the Workplace

Beyond the issue of paid family leave is the case of employed breastfeeding mothers getting support when they do return to work and are still breastfeeding. Breastfeeding is recommended for a year to two (or more) for best benefits, so even if there is paid leave for six months, many mothers of infants will still be breastfeeding when they return to work. In 2017, 65.1% of American mothers with children under six years of age were working outside the home, according to the Bureau of Labor Statistics. Of those employed mothers, 77% were working full time.

Breastfeeding-friendly business practices are slowly improving for mothers working in higher paid jobs, but many lower-income and part-time working mothers do not receive any breastfeeding support from their jobs, meaning the mothers and babies who are most vulnerable in our society get the least breastfeeding support. Many people do not understand that if the breasts get overly full when a mom is not able to breastfeed or pump, it not only puts her at higher risk of plugged ducts and <u>mastitis</u> (breast infection), but it also causes her to lose her milk supply. When a mother's breasts get full and stay full, this sends a signal to the hypothalamus to slow or stop the production of milk. This negative feedback system is called <u>feedback inhibitor of lactation</u>, or FIL.

Especially in the early months of breastfeeding, a mom should not let her breasts get too full if she wants to maintain and build her milk production for her growing baby. However, overly full breasts often happen when a breastfeeding mother works, due to her not being able to take frequent enough pumping breaks at work. This issue of too little time and too few times to pump happens in all kinds of employment, but more so in the kind of jobs where lower-income mothers are employed. I have heard so many stories from my work with breastfeeding/working mothers in WIC about having to forgo pumping at work because there is no space or time to do it at their jobs or they fear losing their jobs if they take too many breaks! The moms I work with often work in fast food, house cleaning, or nail salons, where there is no private, clean place for them to pump! So they start using formula for their babies early, which often leads to an earlier-than-intended <u>weaning</u> (breastfeeding cessation) because their milk production slows and their hungry, growing babies start refusing to breastfeed when the milk comes too little and too slow. As noted before, this demonstrates that for the first six months, breastfeeding mothers need paid leave, then, after the baby has started solids (which is recommended at around six months), returning to work is more feasible as the baby is not reliant only on breast milk. Paid leave for the first six months, then working at a *breastfeeding-friendly job*, would promote breastfeeding equity so all breastfeeding/working mothers can breastfeed for longer for greater benefits.

Following are some examples from my work with WIC families that demonstrate the situations and difficulties mothers have with continuing to breastfeed when returning to work:

Mother #1 complains that she can't pump any milk anymore and has almost completely lost her milk supply after her return to full-time work. She tries to offer her breast to baby when at home, but baby gets fussy due to low milk flow/supply and won't stay at the breast anymore.

Mother #2 states she is using a pump due to breast fullness between feeds, and she wants to start saving milk for her return to work. She has to return at six weeks postpartum and feels sure she will not be able to pump at work, so she is trying to save as much milk as possible to delay and minimize use of formula for her baby.

Mother #3 and I discussed getting breastfeeding off to a good start. She has to return to work in a fast food job at six weeks postpartum, and we discussed trying to continue breastfeeding. She stated she had no place to pump there other than the public bathroom.

Mother #4 was expecting her second baby. She breastfed her first for three months and then weaned when she returned to work. She wanted to breastfeed this second baby for longer. She worked as a manager of a fast food business and asked them about pumping at work. She is worried about taking the time to pump from her busy schedule.

Mother #5 discussed how difficult it is at work to take the time she needed to pump enough, and she had to use a bathroom because there was no other place to pump.

Working Laws and the PUMP Act

There is a *national* law added to a section to the Fair Labor Standards Act that guarantees employed mothers who are paid hourly be allowed to pump milk so they can continue breastfeeding their babies, and that employers should accommodate them with (unpaid) time and a private space to pump. It specifies that the space should not be a bathroom. This national law was passed in 2010 and is called "Break Time for Nursing Mothers." It is associated with the work break time of 15 minutes every four hours, which is not often enough when a mother returns to work while her younger baby is exclusively and frequently breastfeeding. Pumping breaks need to be as often as a baby feeds at breast, and younger babies feed more often than every four hours! This bill also does not apply to salaried employees or employers who have fewer than 50 employees, so it is not comprehensive enough. It is also unworkable for many of my clients who work in fast food establishments, where there are *no* private spaces. Another law covers federal breastfeeding employees, but this affects a very small number of working/breastfeeding mothers. *All* working/breastfeeding mothers need to be covered by legislation in *every* type of job!

In January 2020, the Providing Urgent Maternal Protections (PUMP) for Nursing Mothers Act (S. 3170/H.R. 5592) was proposed to Congress to strengthen the 2010 "Break Time for Nursing Mothers" Law. The PUMP Act would:

- Ensure that *all* breastfeeding employees are covered by the Break Time law.
- Create a clear mechanism for holding employers accountable when they do not comply.

PUMP Act will extend the previous protections for working/breastfeeding mothers to around 9 more million breastfeeding workers, including nurses, teachers, engineers, and other salaried workers. The PUMP Act will also give employers more clarity about breastfeeding employees' needs regarding breaks to express/pump their milk for their babies. This legislation is needed, as the old legislation is vague, inadequate, and confusing. I hope the PUMP Act is passed into law!

Businesses who support breastfeeding moms with breastfeeding-friendly work policies enjoy better productivity and loyalty from their working/breastfeeding mothers. Also, businesses that provide health insurance to their breastfeeding employees' families enjoy lower health insurance costs due to the better health of the employees' babies. Another benefit is that mothers who breastfeed fully and for longer usually have longer time between pregnancies, which benefits employers when they have less frequent maternity leaves. Businesses that provide paid leave and breastfeeding-friendly policies get a substantial payback when they support their breastfeeding employees, so it is in their best interests to support breastfeeding/working employees!

The Legal Case for Breastfeeding Protection and Support

I've discussed federal laws regarding pumping at work, but the United States does not have any other legislation regarding the most basic rights involved in breastfeeding. For example, there is no national law regarding breastfeeding in public spaces. Breastfeeding mothers are often harassed and persecuted for breastfeeding in public. Breastfeeding has been considered "indecent exposure" by many, and mothers are told to go to the bathroom to breastfeed or are banished from public spaces. Security guards are notorious for admonishing and harassing mothers for breastfeeding in public! In St. Louis, one mother who was breastfeeding in her car in a parking lot had the police called on her and was even arrested for breastfeeding in public! Eventually the charges were dropped, but she and her baby had to endure being arrested. Another mom I knew was barred from completing her business at the City Hall due to trying to breastfeed her baby while there.

Breastfeeding advocates in many states took initiatives to get state laws passed to clarify that breastfeeding is not indecent exposure and should be legal wherever a mother and baby have a right to be in public or private spaces. This led to state-by-state legislation on breastfeeding rights in public and slowly, over almost three decades, resulted in variable degrees of protection for breastfeeding in public. It's really astonishing that such a basic human right has so little and so variable protection!

Florida and New York were the first states to pass breastfeeding legislation in the early 1990s, and other states followed, with 2018 being the year the last of the states passed breastfeeding legislation clarifying that breastfeeding in public is legal. Each state has *variable* laws now regarding breastfeeding in public and breastfeeding support. California, Illinois, and New York have some of the most comprehensive breastfeeding support laws, covering such things as jury duty, childcare, employment, pumping at work, lactation stations to accommodate mothers in airports and other public buildings, etc. Some other states have only one piece of breastfeeding legislation that guarantees a mother's right to breastfeed in public. Missouri, my home state, has a law with the word "discretion" in it: "Notwithstanding any other provision of law to the contrary, a mother may, *with discretion*, breast-feed her child or express breast milk in any public or private location where the mother is otherwise authorized to be." This word, "discretion" is confusing and shouldn't be there—whose discretion does it mean?—but breastfeeding advocates in Missouri, including myself, were unable to get that word removed. Besides, there is so much more to the legal issue of breastfeeding than just breastfeeding in public spaces.

The issue with each state having their own distinct and limited breastfeeding legislation is that there are too many differences and we are too mobile and interconnected a society for such variability in laws about a basic right such as breastfeeding. We need a comprehensive *national* law regarding anything to do with breastfeeding. It is a basic human right! A law protecting and supporting a woman's unique ability to breastfeed could be modeled after the laws regarding disability protections, accommodations, and support. We need federal legislation such as an "American Breastfeeding Act," similar to the Americans with Disabilities Act, that would prevent discrimination, require accommodations and support, and, importantly, legislate funding for this to happen. This legislation would be based on an *ability* (to breastfeed) instead of a disability though. Of course, the choice to breastfeed or not should be built into the law, and the law could be used more broadly to support parental care and the nurturing of a young infant in the first year of life, no matter how the infant is fed or which parent does the majority of the daily care of that infant.

Comprehensive federal legislation regarding a national paid family leave for six months, comprehensive legislation regarding breastfeeding/working, and legislation covering breastfeeding rights in *all* social domains for *all* mothers are desperately needed in America!

Other Health Outcomes as Related to Breastfeeding/CDC Maps

Breastfeeding rates are understandably lower among certain groups and communities, such as low-income and undersupported mothers who return to marginal employment situations not conducive to breastfeeding. Lower breastfeeding rates in these groups relate to higher infant mortality rates and health and social inequities that plague these same communities. This is very evident with regards to the southern US and among African American communities. In addition to low breastfeeding rates, these populations suffer from a higher incidence of more serious health and social problems. CDC data and maps clearly illustrate the geographical and socioeconomic patterns of diseases, poverty, social ills, and low breastfeeding rates. They all tend to overlap, and although this does not imply causation, it does highly imply correlation.

The following are some examples of specific CDC maps for the issues that I have discussed as related to breastfeeding: obesity, diabetes, infant mortality, race, breast cancer, and poverty. There are many more CDC maps that also show higher illness incidence for heart disease, high blood pressure, strokes, cancers, and other major illnesses that also correlate with the lower rates of breastfeeding. These maps are indicative that low breastfeeding rates correlate with higher illness and death rates, lost productivity, and higher health care and social costs in the US. Conversely, higher breastfeeding rates correlate where breastfeeding support and resources are greater and with better health indicators and lower illness and mortality rates.

WIC keeps breastfeeding rates on every mother and infant involved in WIC, but many mothers do not report accurate breastfeeding status because they want to get more formula on their food package to save up for later need. This leads to inaccuracy in the WIC breastfeeding data, but at least WIC does attempt to assess and document breastfeeding rates on all mothers and infants involved in WIC.

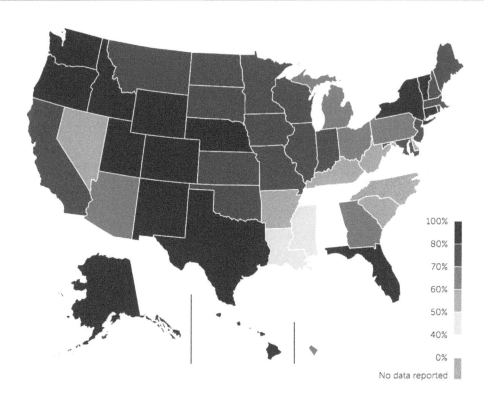

WIC Breastfeeding Initiation Rates by State (2018):

100%
80%
70%
60%
50%
40%
0%
No data reported

The map above shows breastfeeding initiation rates as reported by WIC. These rates only indicate the start of breastfeeding, so they include an unknown number of babies who only breastfed while in the hospital or only for a few days. This initiation data is not as valuable as measurements of breastfeeding continuation rates, such as those estimated in the following four maps generated from National Immunization Survey responses.

Estimated breastfeeding rates are based on the National Immunization Survey, a random phone survey of less than 1% of parents of 19– to 35-month-old infants. Infants living in the Southeast have lower breastfeeding continuation rates and are less likely to be breastfed for six months than infants living in other areas of the country.

Percentages of infants who **ever** breastfeed (2016):

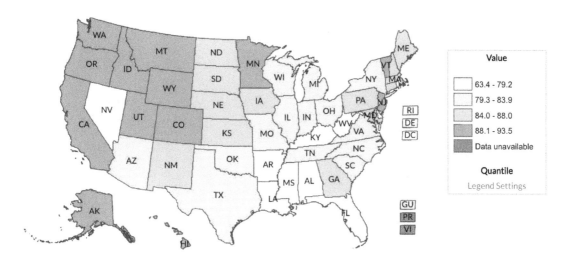

Percentages of infants who breastfeed **exclusively** through **three** months (2016):

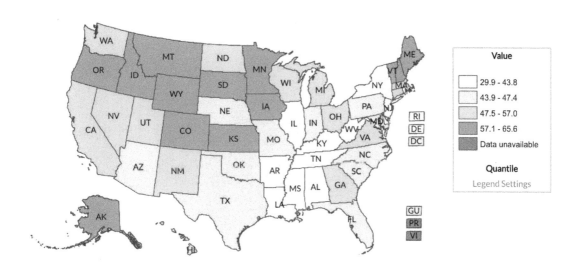

Percentages of infants who breastfeed **exclusively** through **six** months:

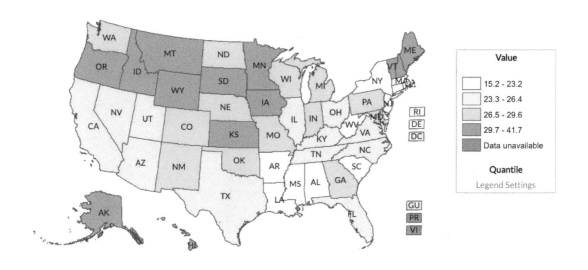

Percentages of infants who breastfed for **twelve** months, **exclusively or partially:**

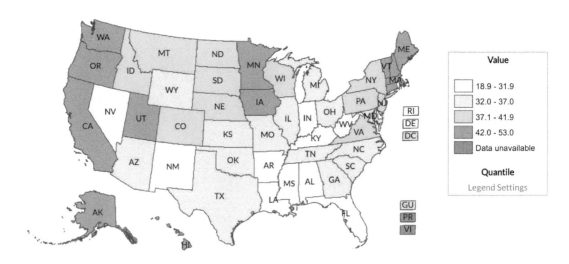

Infant mortality rates correlate with lower breastfeeding rates in Southeast America:

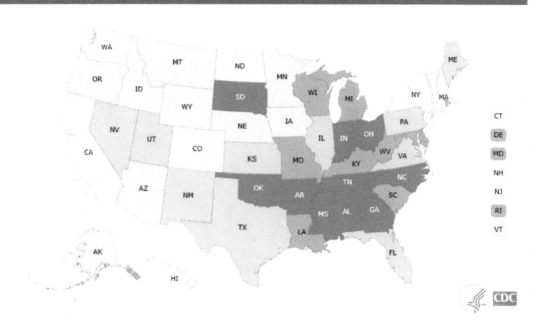

Infant Mortality Rates by State, 2017

Death Rates[1]

United States 5.8

- 3.7 - 4.6
- 4.6 - 5.7
- 5.7 - 6.1
- 6.2 - 7.1
- 7.1 - 8.6

[1]The number of infant deaths per 1,000 live births.

Infant Mortality Rates by Race and Ethnicity, 2016

The following rates show the highest infant mortality among African Americans, who also have the lowest breastfeeding rates and highest breastfeeding barriers. There is a higher ratio of African Americans in the southeastern area of the US, correlating with lower breastfeeding rates in those states, as noted. Sadly, African Americans are still being affected by the history and effects of slavery and civil rights deprivations, with ensuing higher rates of poverty and social disadvantages. These disadvantages have led to lower breastfeeding rates and worse health outcomes among the African American community in America.

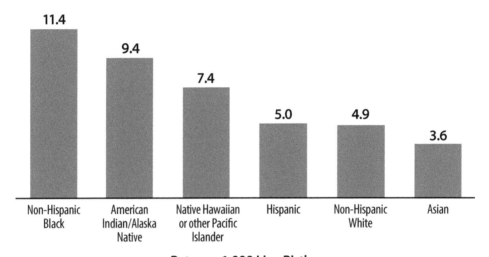

Rate per 1,000 Live Births

Higher obesity rates correlate with the lower breastfeeding rates in the US. The prevalence of obesity in the US remains much higher than our National Health goals of 14.5% among youth and 30.5% among adults. Obesity has become our most costly preventable illness, surpassing tobacco-related illness. The medical care costs of obesity in the United States are high: these costs are estimated from $150 billion to over $200 billion annually, or nearly 20% of annual medical spending in the United States. Obesity leads to many other health-related problems, such as diabetes, as well.

Prevalence of obesity in the US in 2018 (among adults, self-reported):

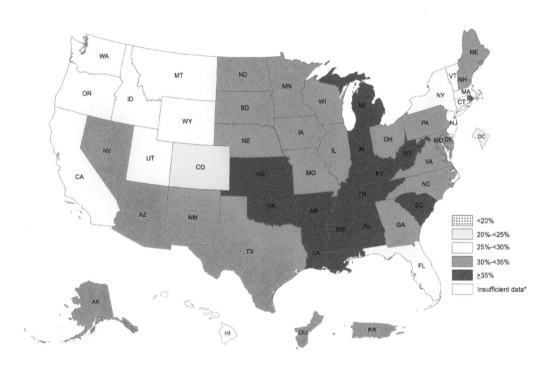

Source: Behavioral Risk Factor Surveillance System
*Sample size <50, the relative standard error (dividing the standard error by the prevalence) ≥30%, or no data in a specific year.

County-Level Distribution of Diagnosed Diabetes Among US Adults Aged 20 or Older, 2013

States where diabetes prevalence is the highest (the "diabetes belt") also have the lowest breastfeeding rates, as seen in the previous maps on breastfeeding incidence (2018):

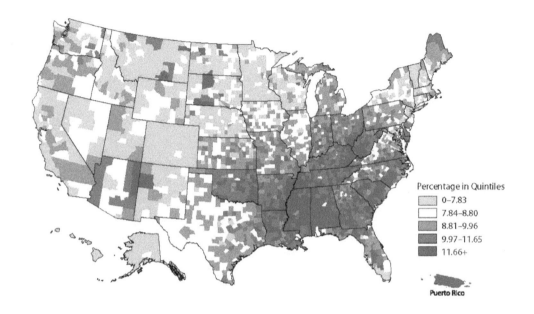

The 1950s was the era when the breastfeeding rates bottomed out at an estimated rate of 15% to 20%, and continuation rates were minimal. It is very telling that the rates of diabetes have climbed since that time of the lowest breastfeeding rates as people who were the "least breastfed" come of the age where metabolic illness shows its greatest impact.

Rates of diabetes incidence are just beginning to slow in their increases more recently with younger people. Might that be due to higher breastfeeding rates of recent years?

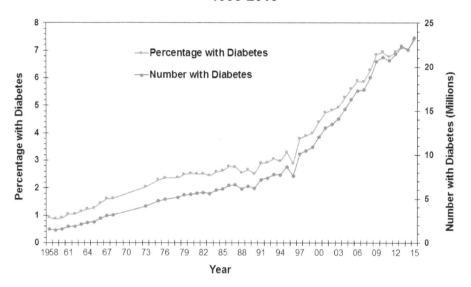

Number and Percentage of U.S. Population with Diagnosed Diabetes, 1958-2015

CDC's Division of Diabetes Translation. United States Diabetes Surveillance System available at http://www.cdc.gov/diabetes/data

Breastfeeding also reduces the risk of breast cancer.

Breast cancer mortality:

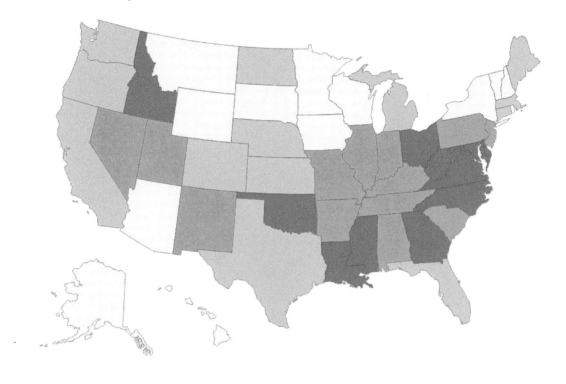

Rate per 100,000 women

| 15.6 - 18.1 | 18.3 - 19.8 | 20.0 - 21.3 | 21.5 - 25.3 |

According to Pew Research Center data, the greatest federal spending per state GDP are in the southern states. Mississippi was the recipient of the greatest amount of federal dollars, which amounted to a third of its GDP in 2014.

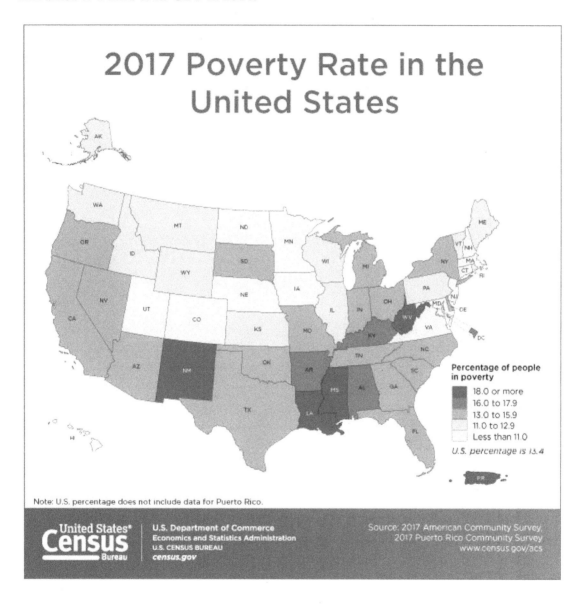

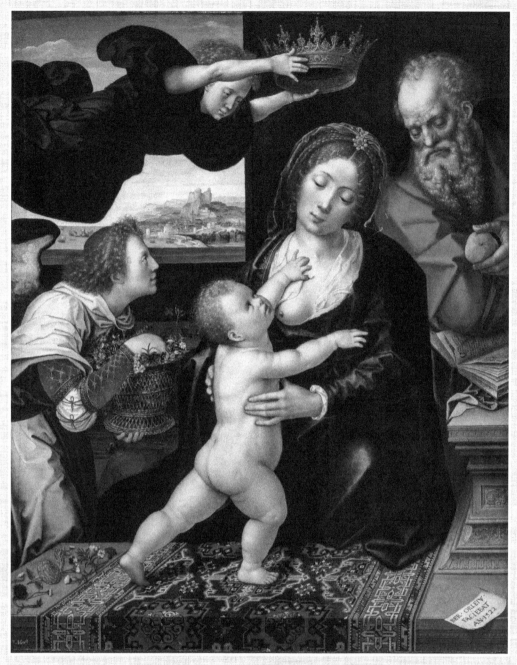

Bernard van Orley, *La Sagrada Familia* (*The Holy Family*), A.D. 1522—depicting
the value of and support for the breastfeeding mother!

Summary

When babies get the best start in life, they have a much better chance to thrive and grow up to be healthy and productive. When the work of breastfeeding is assessed, valued, and supported as it needs to be by our country and institutions, women will be recognized for their unique contribution to their baby's health and well-being. Mothers supported by paid family leave and having their jobs held will not lose career status while they bear, birth, and breastfeed the future citizens of our country. When all mothers and babies receive this support regardless of their education, expertise, race, background, job type, or income, this will improve gender, social, and health equity in America, and our health data maps will look very different when breastfeeding prevails in all the United States' communities!

I have covered the importance of breastfeeding for babies, moms, families, communities, the environment, our health care and economic systems, and society at large. Yes, humans are omnivorous and are able to survive on less ideal foods, such as formula and other highly processed foods. Our ability to be omnivorous and eat a wide variety of types of foods is partly why humans are the "top mammals." We will always need some use of formulas (or, more desirably, banked human milk) for some babies when breastfeeding is not possible or chosen, but there is so much evidence that supports breastfeeding as the finest method of feeding and nurturing a baby. So why haven't we as a country done more to support this potent public health tool and the women who do the work of breastfeeding? Why are we not even accurately assessing and documenting breastfeeding practices and statistics on *all* babies? Why are we one of just a few countries to not have a national paid family leave? Why do we have so few human milk banks if we are the richest country? Why are there not more lactation professionals to meet the growing need and demand for their services in America? Why are there not more comprehensive *national* laws and policies protecting breastfeeding mothers and babies in America? Why do we not have a comprehensive health insurance coverage as a right so all moms and babies can get the breastfeeding support and treatments that will help them successfully breastfeed?

Our lack of recognition, documentation, and support of the uniquely womanly work of breastfeeding implicates our paternalistic, capitalistic, and medicalized tendencies to value profit over health. We have a tertiary medical care system profiting from human illness rather than a primary health care system striving to prevent illness. We allow corporations to profit and to promote their formulas through our maternity care system, free samples, and free advertising of their inferior product. We refuse to adopt the World Health Organization "Code," which dictates the marketing of breast milk substitutes and restricts formula promotion and marketing. At the 2018 World Health Assembly, the United States Health and Human Services even tried to influence other countries to allow formula to be more freely advertised by lessening the protections afforded by "the Code" so that we could more easily sell more formula to those countries.

We heavily subsidize WIC for formula distribution and don't dedicate enough funding for breastfeeding support and care in WIC. We refuse to adopt a national paid leave policy that would allow all mothers to spend more time at home with their newborns, getting breastfeeding and parenting off to a better start before they return to work. We place all the responsibility, work, and time of breastfeeding upon the mothers' shoulders even though we *ALL* benefit from the work of breastfeeding as a society.

Our neglect to give the needed social, economic, legislative, and health care supports that our mothers and babies need for breastfeeding success has helped us to become a *tertiary care* society. In this regard, we have surrendered our self-health powers to industries that use their money and influence to discourage our government from enacting laws and policies that would support breastfeeding but would decrease their profits. This results in the formula and pharmaceutical companies having undue influence over how our babies in America are fed and nurtured.

Women are still not enjoying equal rights, recognition, pay, and support for our unique contributions to American society and our work in bearing, birthing, and breastfeeding the future citizens of this country! Just as we aren't going to reap the many benefits that breastfeeding has to offer from token breastfeeding, we aren't going to reap the many benefits from token support of breastfeeding.

The following is a summary of the "ingredients" that I have discussed in this book. These ingredients are needed for a "recipe" for effective support of breastfeeding mothers and babies in America. These recommendations for a *recipe of breastfeeding support*, if enacted, will have far-reaching benefits for all of American society because *breastfeeding, and its support, is* a *key health ingredient* that is needed for equitable health and well-being in America!

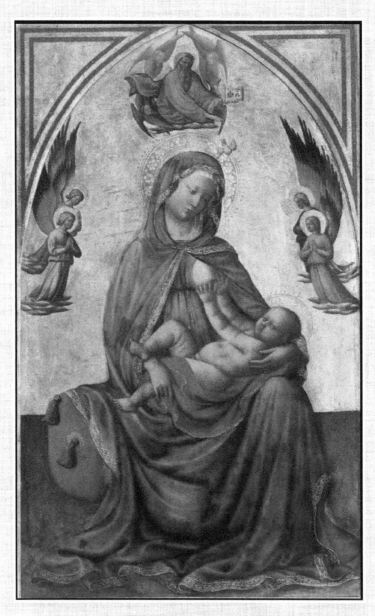

Masolino da Panicale, *Madonna and Child*, circa AD 1435.

Recommended Breastfeeding Support Ingredients for the United States

- Adopt and enforce the WHO "Code" (the International Code of Marketing of Breast-milk Substitutes) at the national level.

- Assess and document accurate, real-time breastfeeding statuses on medical charts of all babies at every well-baby visit. This data should be compiled by the Centers for Disease Control to report more detailed and accurate breastfeeding statistics and analysis. This would give exclusive, partial, and continuation breastfeeding statistics and would emphasize the importance of breastfeeding by just asking the questions! *The question that gets asked gets attention, and what gets counted counts in our health care system!*

- Establish a national policy for paid family leave for a minimum of six months. Since six months of exclusive breastfeeding is the standard recommendation, our national paid leave should cover at least six months. Paid time off after the birth of a baby will provide a breastfeeding mother time and support to get breastfeeding off to a better start and will help her reach her breastfeeding goals and provide other dose-related benefits from breastfeeding. Paid leave could be used by fathers when it is a family decision to have the mother work and the father stay at home with the baby. Paid leave would have a positive impact for our families and communities far beyond the issue of breastfeeding.

- Require all maternal and infant care services to be breastfeeding/baby friendly and provide government funding to help with the training and certification for this effort. Currently, only 26.8% of births in the US occur in breastfeeding/baby-friendly hospitals. Baby-Friendly USA should also expand its reach to other medical issues that cause breastfeeding difficulties, like the overuse of IV fluids, overuse of Pitocin, and circumcision on the second day of life before breastfeeding is well established.

- Require as part of Baby-Friendly that all RN staff working in labor and delivery become IBCLC certified to better serve their clients with breastfeeding needs.

- Increase state and national funding for breastfeeding/lactation education in these three areas:

  #1: Funding for more training and educational programs to increase the number of breastfeeding support providers, including IBCLCs, Certified Lactation Counselors (CLCs), peer counselors, and others. We especially need more women of color to become IBCLCs, CLCs, and peer counselors for breastfeeding equity! African American mothers have the lowest breastfeeding rates due to increased barriers to breastfeeding. Currently, almost all IBCLCs are white, and that needs to change to represent and better serve the greater diversity in America!

  #2: Expand breastfeeding education, services, and support to those areas and communities not currently served or not adequately served and to those communities with higher breastfeeding barriers as evidenced by low breastfeeding rates.

  #3: Increase basic lactation education for other health care professionals: MDs, RNs, RDs, PTs, and other health care providers who work with mothers and babies.

- Enact legislation and policy to protect breastfeeding as a natural resource, similar to such policies enacted to protect environmental resources.

- Enact comprehensive national laws and policies concerning breastfeeding protection and support. We are a mobile and interconnected country, and because breastfeeding is such a basic public health issue, federal laws and policies regarding breastfeeding are better than state-by-state laws and policies. Currently, every state has different laws about breastfeeding; this is too confusing. Federal laws and policies regarding breastfeeding rights would alleviate the discrepancies in the current state breastfeeding laws and policies. All the laws and policies regarding breastfeeding in public, health care system support, protection for breastfeeding, paid leave, jury duty relief, lactation consultant education funding, insurance coverage, and breastfeeding statistics need to be comprehensive and provide *national* coverage for this basic human right—the right to breastfeed.

- Provide comprehensive insurance coverage for all breastfeeding mothers and babies that fully covers health and lactation services and supplies without deductibles or copays. A national health insurance coverage such as "Medicare for All" would cover all people, provide comprehensive coverage for primary care including breastfeeding needs/lactation services, would be affordable, and would be a lot less confusing!

- Increase milk banking. There are only 25 milk banks in the US. Other countries have far more: Brazil has over 200 milk banks, and there are 223 across Europe. We need human milk banks in at least every city that has a NICU.

- Fund and perform more research into breastfeeding and breast milk. Katie Hinde points out so well in her TED talk that the National Institutes of Health has more research about coffee, wine, tomatoes, and cow's milk than human milk and breastfeeding! A telling gender discrepancy is the fact that there is twice as much research about erectile dysfunction than about breastfeeding.

- Conduct a nationwide economic analysis comparing the costs of breastfeeding versus formula feeding/not breastfeeding. This analysis should include increased health care costs, product manufacturing, price, advertising, transportation, storage, and environmental and social costs of formula feeding. This analysis will be easier and more accurate if we have well-documented breastfeeding statistics on every baby in the health care system.

- Recognize the important economic value of breastfeeding by including it in the USA's GDP to recognize the work involved in mothers' breastfeeding and as the rationale for funding devoted to breastfeeding support measures. Failure to account for mothers' milk production in GDP and economic data renders our mothers' work breastfeeding invisible. This lack of an economic value for breastfeeding stymies programs and policies that protect and support women to breastfeed. When breastfeeding is counted and assigned a value, then it can be better protected from competing market pressures.

- Gradually decrease subsidies for dairy farmers' and pharmaceutical companies' production of formula and redirect these funds to increase subsidies for breastfeeding mothers and babies. These subsidies should include paid family leave, expansion of breastfeeding services, increased funding for health care delivery systems to become breastfeeding/baby-friendly, funding more research on breastfeeding, and subsidizing breastfeeding products. Some of this redirected money could also be used for more research into improvement of the formula product. We will always need some formula for babies and mothers who can't or choose not to breastfeed, and, at the very least, they deserve a better product! We also need to fund more human milk banks and could be using our tax money to establish and support them instead of continuing to subsidize formula. Human milk, and breastfeeding mothers, need our subsidies more than formula!

- WIC should gradually extricate itself from serving the formula industry by increasing breastfeeding services and benefits and by paying full market price for formula (following "the Code"), which would lead to a gradual decrease of formula to WIC participants, while increasing breastfeeding support and better food packages for the breastfeeding mother.

- Fund public service announcements and programming (broadcast and online) educating the public about the importance of breastfeeding. Do not allow formula manufacturers to negatively influence this, as they have done in the past. These announcements or short programs would help send strong and positive messages to the public and, over time, help change perceptions and increase acceptance of breastfeeding as the norm in our American culture.

- Officially recognize and honor the founders of La Leche League, the breastfeeding support organization. The founders of La Leche League deserve a Nobel Peace Prize and other national awards for their enduring service and commitment to mothers and babies by offering volunteer breastfeeding support for more than 63 years. Of the seven founders (Mary Ann Kerwin, Viola Brennan Lennon, Betty Wagner Spandikow, Edwina Hearn Froehlich, Mary White, Mary Ann Cahill, and Marian Leonard Tompson), only the last two are still alive. The time to recognize them is long overdue, and the fact that they have not been awarded is a prime example of the gender discrimination in the Nobel Foundation (since the first Nobel Prize was awarded in 1901, women have won it 54 times, men 919 times).

Immediate Action Steps Mothers and Others Can Take

1. When you have a baby, please give breastfeeding a good effort! It is work, can be hard, and involves a strong commitment, but do it for yourself, not only for your baby! Breastfeeding is important for your health and maternal empowerment, as well as your baby's health. Even if you can't exclusively breastfeed, try to partially breastfeed, as that has benefits also. Breastfeeding is not an all-or-nothing issue, and some mothers have too many barriers to breastfeed fully. We are seeing epigenetic changes in American women from our long history (many generations) of non-breastfeeding (metabolic syndrome, obesity, diabetes, fertility problems), and these conditions make it harder to breastfeed and can cause low milk supply. This is nature's "do it or lose it" message—breastfeed or lose the ability to! If we want to continue to enjoy our breasts filling out sweaters, then we need to use them to fill up our babies' tummies! Please seek and ***demand the support*** you need to help you continue breastfeeding! Consumer demand is important to driving change in America!

2. Safely donate or share your breast milk if you have plenty. Become a milk donor. Milk banks are always in need of donated breast milk! Milk depots (drop-off sites for sending in milk to a milk bank) make it easier to donate pumped breast milk and are getting established in some cities. Demand more milk banks in the US so babies other than the most fragile can receive human milk when their mothers cannot or choose not to breastfeed.

3. Milk sharing is an ancient practice among mothers, and although it is not without risks, there are risks from formula feeding, and these risks need to be considered in the infant-feeding choice. Safe milk sharing guidelines are available from the Academy of Breastfeeding Medicine (see the Notes).

4. Get involved with La Leche League or another breastfeeding support group so you can receive support and camaraderie from peers. Start a breastfeeding support group in your area if there is not one that meets your needs. Mother-to-mother (peer) breastfeeding support is very potent, and we need it in addition to professional support. Also, individually supporting other family members or friends on their breastfeeding journeys is an invaluable gift.

5. If you are so inclined, and especially if you work with mothers and babies in your professional capacity, think about becoming certified as a lactation consultant, as the lactation field is underpopulated, underrecognized, and underfunded. We need more women of color, more cultures, and more ages enriching our profession. If you work in a health care capacity, ask that your organization sponsor and fund the education you need to help you get certified. Advocate for more educational opportunities and educational programs to meet the growing need for lactation professionals, and federal funding to support this growing need.

6. If you are a partner to a breastfeeding mother, give the support that is needed that you have in your power to give. Educate yourself on how to be a breastfeeding supporter in your family. Don't think this is just a mothering issue, as breastfeeding success benefits all. Don't be afraid to speak out about the importance of breastfeeding support, as it goes way beyond just being a mother's or woman's issue!

7. Join and form alliances between breastfeeding coalitions, other family/child coalitions, and service providers in America! How much more powerful and effective it would be for more organizations and coalitions to join forces promoting/supporting breastfeeding. Breastfeeding deserves much more attention and support from all sectors of society, and increased success with breastfeeding helps to ameliorate many other problems addressed by other coalitions/ organizations.

8. As breastfeeding health care consumers, you can ask that your breastfeeding status get documented at every well-baby and maternal visit on the health care record. Your work breastfeeding deserves to be documented! If you work in the medical care system, advocate for adding the breastfeeding assessment questions to the electronic health record (EHR) for use at the well-baby/immunization visits at your health care sites, and document breastfeeding status at every well-baby visit.

9. If you feel like your health care provider/system/insurance or employer did not give you the breastfeeding education, support, and/or service you feel you were entitled to, and your breastfeeding experience was hampered or thwarted, then you might think about a lawsuit against the persons or system! I know that would take a lot of money, time, and effort, so many would not be able to pursue this route, but sometimes it takes lawsuits for our systems to change. One example of discrimination that occurs is when a health care provider does not give breastfeeding education and encouragement to a pregnant woman due to that woman's culture, race, age, or other characteristic.

10. Write letters to legislative representatives asking for the US to enact the World Health Organization's International Code of Marketing of Breast-milk Substitutes, as described previously; for the increase of national funding for lactation education and services; for paid family leave and Medicare for All or expanded Medicaid; and better national laws and policies to protect breastfeeding. Expanding the protection of breastfeeding laws to the federal level instead of state by state is important so that the laws will be uniform and comprehensive throughout the country and would protect all American breastfeeding mothers and babies. Any breastfeeding federal law should be at least as comprehensive as the most comprehensive breastfeeding law at the state level.

11. Request a breastfeeding stamp in America to increase awareness of the importance of breastfeeding and to raise money to promote breastfeeding in America, the way the breast cancer stamp has been utilized. Ask art museums to bring back breastfeeding art to represent the fact that most mothers are choosing to breastfeed. Art serves an important function reflecting and encouraging what is healthy!

12. Organize a national call-in-sick-for-paid-family-leave day scheduled on a work day. Promote it through social media as well as family organizations and coalitions devoted to mothers and babies. If even 30% of the non-emergency American workforce were to call in sick on the proposed day, it would send a strong message advocating for national paid family leave! Or if even 30% of the childbearing women in America went on a *birth strike*, that would send a powerful message to our country that we do have power to withhold birthing future citizens if we don't get paid family leave! Think of the effect that would have on our economy and society at large: the less utilized labor and delivery suites in hospitals; the less busy OB doctors

and pediatricians; the less products, services, and medicines sold for moms and babies; the less future workers in our country! America's birth rate has been rapidly declining and is now around 1.7 per family. Lower birth rates combined with lower immigration equals fewer future workers to support our aging population. America needs healthy babies and also needs to provide mothers with recognition and support for their unique ability to bear, birth, and breastfeed them! I hope that the National Organization of Women and other institutions concerned with women's rights will take up this issue.

13. Please refrain from the divisive "mommy wars," as that pits women against women and divides our power and effectiveness. Breastfeeding support encompasses supports and systems that benefit all mothers and women. Breastfeeding is not an all-or-nothing issue, and our work toward the issues I have discussed in this book will benefit all mothers, children, and families, regardless of how much or how long or even if they don't breastfeed.

14. Vote for and help elect women to legislative offices who understand the importance of breastfeeding and will advocate and work for laws, policies, paid leave, and health insurance coverage to increase breastfeeding and family support in America. Women are not well represented in state and federal legislative offices. Women represent only 24% of those in Congress and 28.7 % in state legislatures. We have never had a woman president in the US, yet women are over 50% of the population in America! It is time this changed, and 2020 holds promise for women being elected in greater numbers and gaining power on important issues such as breastfeeding support in America! How about a woman in the oval office?!

Final Statement

Breastfeeding is the optimal, bioactive *product and process* to feed, nurture, comfort, grow, protect, and immunize our precious babies. It is a ready-on-demand system, requires minimal material resources, keeps infants and mothers together, reduces illness and suffering, enhances the pleasure of being a mother and a baby when it is going well, is self-produced and empowering for the mother, and reduces reliance on costly for-profit systems. It inspires mothers to be more intimately involved with their children and enhances bonds in relationships not only between mother and baby, but also mother-to-mother and between families and supporters. Breastfeeding is alive, dynamic, and specific to each baby (a mom's special recipe for her special baby); it is the first and freshest "slow food," which establishes a healthy microbiome in the baby's gut and a healthy eating style; it comes in flavors influenced by the foods a mother eats; it is a mom's multipurpose tool for nurturing and comforting her baby; and, importantly, breastfeeding comes in self-producing, empowering, reusable, environmentally friendly, and attractive packaging and is delivered in a warm and loving embrace!

When will America wake up and realize breastfeeding is a most potent and worthy public health tool, count it as important work of mothering, and support our breastfeeding moms and babies as they really need and deserve to be supported? Maybe our recent worries about coronavirus and its greater morbidity among people with comorbidities will wake our country up to this important issue of breastfeeding and breastfeeding support, which is seriously needed and deserved. Breastfeeding is an important ingredient for the health and well-being of moms, babies, and our country, and *support given to breastfeeding mothers* is the best recipe for affordable and equitable health care and better health and well-being in America!

To make this serious subject more colorful, I've included some pictures of breastfeeding art and breastfeeding stamps from around the world, and in the spirit of a "recipe" book, I've included a list of recommended "ingredients" needed to make the recipe of proper breastfeeding support in America!

I hope you have found this book worthy of your attention. Thank you for taking an interest in the worthy subject of breastfeeding! I hope some of my ideas and "ingredients" get used in our national and communal "recipe" for breastfeeding support in America!

—*Erin L. O'Reilly*

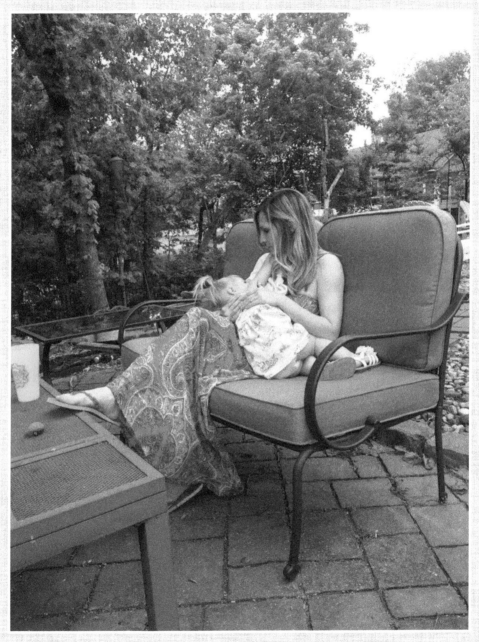

Theresa and Madeline Nicholaus affectionately breastfeeding.

Acknowledgments

Writing a book is harder and has taken a lot longer than I thought, but I have learned so much!

None of this would have been possible without my editor, Andrew Doty, who had to not only guide me in writing and publishing a book, but also in all the tech stuff necessary to know for writing a book. He was the first editor I called, and I'm glad I called him! He had all the connections with others needed to get this book ready for self-publishing, including Peggy Nehmen, who has played an important, and very helpful, role in getting the visual aspects of this book taken care of so expertly. I'm very appreciative of their work, skills, and talents! Karen Tucker and Lisa Ashpole, my copyeditor and proofreader, also played important roles in this process.

I want to thank BJ Diamond, my sister-in-law, for her preliminary editing when I first started writing this book. I'm also grateful to Kelly West and Robert Perks, and their daughter Eilah, for the front-cover photo, as well as their photographer, Gabriella Marks. And I'm thankful to Theresa Nickolaus and her husband Mike for the photo of Theresa and their daughter, Madeline, at the end of the book.

I also want to give appreciation to my husband, Jay Diamond, who has listened to me about this book for a good many years and has given valuable feedback! Of course, I am also grateful to Jesse Diamond, my son, who inspired me to breastfeed, which led me down this path of breastfeeding support and also to writing this book. As a young child of a breastfeeding supporter, he attended many La Leche League meetings, had to wait while I counseled breastfeeding mothers on many phone calls, and endured riding in his mom's car with all my breastfeeding slogan bumper stickers!

Glossary

Acute health: Short-term health, in contrast to chronic health.

Affordable Care Act (ACA): The comprehensive health care reform law enacted in March 2010 ("Obamacare"). The law's goals: make affordable health insurance available to more people.

Apgar score: A measure of the physical condition of a newborn infant obtained by adding points (2, 1, or 0) for heart rate, respiratory function, muscle tone, response to stimulation, and skin color; a score of 10 represents the best possible condition.

Baby-Friendly Hospital Initiative (BFHI): A worldwide program of the World Health Organization and UNICEF, launched in 1991 following the adoption of the Innocenti Declaration on breastfeeding promotion.

Bioactive: Affecting living organisms.

Bioavailability: The degree to which nutrients, probiotics, hormones, and neurochemicals are available for absorption and utilization in the body.

Birth strike: A social action by women for the purpose of getting paid family leave and other benefits for mothers and babies. It is already happening in America, so why not actually call it what it is?! Jenny Brown identified this term in her book named *Birth Strike*.

Breast milk: Milk produced in the human breast of the mother for her infant. Human milk contains living and dynamic nutrients that are suited for infant requirements for development, growth, and a healthy immune system. Human milk also contains immunologic agents and other compounds that act against viruses, bacteria, and parasites and protect against chronic illnesses later in life.

Breastfeeding: When a baby feeds directly from a breast, as opposed to consuming pre-pumped breast milk (breast milk feeding).

Breastfeeding goals: The breastfeeding recommendations are to fully breastfeed a baby for the first six months of their life and to continue partially breastfeeding the baby until they are one year old, while also introducing solid foods into the baby's diet after the first six months. Individual and national breastfeeding goals are based on these recommendations.

Breastfeeding Report Card: The CDC's biannual estimate and report of breastfeeding statistics.

Breastfeeding-friendly: This describes a place or situation that is welcoming to breastfeeding moms and babies, supports them, and tries to reduce breastfeeding barriers. Also referred to as baby-friendly as in the Baby-Friendly Hospital Initiative (BFHI).

Centers for Disease Control and Prevention (CDC): Federal health care agency charged with protecting public health related to diseases, injuries, and disabilities in the US and internationally. The CDC makes health recommendations based on the data it collects.

Certified Lactation Counselor (CLC): A health care professional who works in breastfeeding counseling and management in the community. This certification is granted by the Academy of Lactation Policy and Practice, Inc. It's easier and less involved to become a CLC than an IBCLC. Many hospitals require an IBCLC to work in the health care setting.

Chronic illness: An illness that lasts three months or longer and can't be cured by medicine. Three of the top chronic diseases are heart disease, cancer, and diabetes, which are leading causes of disability and death and health care costs.

Circumcision: Circumcision surgery removes the foreskin that covers and protects the tip of the penis. It is usually done on the second day of life before a newborn leaves the hospital.

Direct breastfeeding: See breastfeeding.

Division of Family Services (DFS): A government agency under the Department of Health and Human Services dedicated to providing assistance to and monitoring the safety of children and families. The names of these agencies vary by state and may be referred to as the Department of Social Services, Department of Children and Family Services, Administration for Children and Families, or other names.

Dose-related benefits: The greater extent and longer duration of breastfeeding, the greater the benefits for moms, babies, families, and society.

Doula: A trained and certified supporter for the laboring or postpartum mother. This is a nonmedical caregiver who is well versed in comfort and self/partner-help techniques such as massage, positioning, relaxation, music, and other comfort modalities. Doulas are also often trained to help with basic breastfeeding support and many are CLC certified as well.

Epigenetic: Something that affects a cell, organ, or living entity without directly changing its DNA. An indirect influence on the genome through the life experiences and developmental processes.

Exclusive breastfeeding: Also referred to as "fully breastfeeding," this means a baby is only receiving breast milk for nourishment, except for vitamins or medications, and is not receiving any formula or other milks.

Failure to thrive: A situation in which a child is considered undernourished and does not meet recommended standards of growth.

Feedback inhibitor of lactation (FIL): An ingredient in breast milk that, if the breast is unemptied, sends a negative signal to downregulate the production of breast milk.

Formula: A for-profit, commercially prepared breast milk substitute formulated in accordance to standards to satisfy the basic nutritional requirements of infants up to between four and six months of age. There are no living cells in formula. It is highly processed and usually uses corn syrup as its main carbohydrate. It is always fortified with iron.

Frenectomy: Clipping of the frenulum.

Fully breastfeeding: Generally regarded as <u>exclusive breastfeeding</u> for six months and continued breastfeeding for six or more months while foods are being introduced.

Gross domestic product (GDP): A measure of the value of economic activity within a country. It is the sum of the market values, or prices, of all final goods and services produced in an economy during a period of time. It is an indicator of the health of a nation's economy.

Health inequities: Unfair and unjust differences in health status, health care, and distribution of health resources between different population groups, arising from the social conditions in which people are born, grow, live, work, and age. Lack of breastfeeding support in different communities are an example of a health inequity.

Incidence: The occurrence, rate, or frequency of something.

Infant and maternal mortality rates: The number of infant deaths from birth to up to 1 year of age per 1000 live births and maternal deaths from pregnancy up to 42 days after a birth per 100,000 births.

International Board Certified Lactation Consultant (IBCLC): Certified by the International Board of Lactation Consultant Examiners, an IBCLC specializes in the clinical management of breastfeeding for mothers and babies. IBCLCs usually work in health care settings but can work in the community.

International Code of Marketing of Breast-milk Substitutes: Also commonly referred to as the "WHO Code" or "the Code," adopted by the World Health Organization in 1981 to limit formula advertising, promotion, and payments or gifts to health workers in order to protect the practice of breastfeeding as a public health measure and reduce infant mortality.

Kangaroo care: A method of caring for a baby that emphasizes the importance of holding the naked or partially dressed child against the bare skin of a parent, typically the mother, for as much as possible each day. Studies have found that skin-to-skin holding stabilizes heart and respiratory rates, improves oxygenation, regulates an infant's body temperature, and conserves a baby's calories.

Key health indicator: A quantifiable and documented characteristic of a population that researchers use as supporting evidence for describing the health of a population. Key health indicators are often used by governments to guide health care policy.

La Leche League (LLL): A breastfeeding support group composed of volunteer mothers, founded by seven mothers in 1956. La Leche League is the oldest and most extensive breastfeeding support group in the world and is considered the world authority on the subject of breastfeeding. The IBCLC profession was started by a La Leche League leader in 1986.

Lactational amenorrhea (LAM): Postnatal infertility that occurs when a woman is amenorrheic (not menstruating) and fully breastfeeding. It usually lasts for a range of three to 24 months and depends on how intensively or fully a mother is breastfeeding her baby. It is due to the breastfeeding hormones keeping the normal menstrual cycle hormones in check. The amount of time LAM lasts indicates the amount of protection against hormonal cancers a woman has received from breastfeeding. In other countries where there is less obesity, it importantly helps to space pregnancies, but in America, with our prevalence of obesity, it does not work as well as a method of birth control. La Leche League mothers who fully breastfeed often use LAM successfully as a method of spacing pregnancies. LAM needs further study, as it is a normal and important health indicator for women!

Lactation professional: A professional breastfeeding specialist trained to teach mothers how to feed their babies at the breast and/or pump. They help women experiencing breastfeeding problems, such as latching difficulties, painful nursing, and low milk production. They can be certified at different levels, depending on their education and experience. The most common examples are peer counselors (PCs), Certified Breastfeeding Educators (CBEs), Certified Lactation Counselors (CLCs), and International Board Certified Lactation Consultants (IBCLCs).

Mastitis: A breast infection that occurs more often when a mother's breasts get too full and the milk quits flowing. Plugged ducts can result in mastitis also.

Metabolic disease/syndrome: A cluster of conditions that result in heart disease, stroke, high blood pressure, obesity, diabetes, and fertility problems. These conditions include high cholesterol, high triglycerides, high blood sugar and insulin resistance, hormonal dysregulation, abdominal fat accumulation, and male pattern balding.

Microbiome: The bacteria, fungi, protozoa, and viruses living inside an organism.

National Immunization Survey (NIS): A survey performed by the CDC to assess man-made immunizations. The survey contains four questions about breastfeeding, which are used to produce the biannual Breastfeeding Report Card.

Neonatal intensive care unit (NICU): A hospital ward that provides intensive care to dangerously ill or premature newborn babies.

Obesity: BMI >30% for adults. BMI takes into account a person's weight and height to gauge total body fat. A person with a BMI of 26 to 27 is about 20% overweight, which carries health risks. A BMI of 30 or higher is considered obese and carries more health risks.

Obstetrics (OB): Medical field focused on pregnancy, childbirth, and the postpartum period.

Partial breastfeeding: In partial breastfeeding, a baby receives formula to supplement breastfeeding. Partial breastfeeding needs to be defined and documented by how much breastfeeding versus formula feeding is being done.

Peer counselor: A mother trained by WIC to help other mothers with breastfeeding concerns.

Pre-eclampsia: A disorder of pregnancy characterized by the onset of high blood pressure over 140/90 consistently and often carries a poor pregnancy outcome for both mother and baby. If left untreated, it can lead to eclampsia in which the mother has seizures, which cuts off the blood flow to the uterus and baby.

Primary care: Health education and promotion and disease prevention that costs the least compared to secondary care and tertiary care. Primary care measures are generally less extreme than other types of care and focus on preventive medicine versus reactive medicine.

Secondary care: Early intervention in an illness to manage or cure it. See also: primary care and tertiary care.

Special Supplemental Nutrition Program for Women, Infants, and Children (WIC): A federal nutritional subsidy program serving pregnant and postpartum/breastfeeding mothers and children up to five years of age.

Tertiary care: Serious illness management, which is often the most costly (and usually very unpleasant) compared to primary care and secondary care, involving surgery, medications, and other medical procedures.

Token breastfeeding: Breastfeeding for a much shorter time than recommended and usually not exclusive. Since the benefits of breastfeeding are dose-related, this means many fewer benefits are experienced from token breastfeeding.

Triple feeding: Breastfeeding, pumping breast milk, and supplementing the baby's feed with either pumped milk or formula.

Vital signs: Measurable variables considered to indicate the state of health or medical condition.

Weaning: The cessation of breastfeeding.

Well-baby visit: A baby's visit to the doctor for primary care, health promotion, and immunizations.

WIC: See: Special Supplemental Nutrition Program for Women, Infants, and Children.

World Health Organization (WHO): An agency of the United Nations concerned with international public health.

Notes

For more resources, updated regularly, visit ErinLOReilly.com.

INTRODUCTION:
The CDC's Healthy People Objectives can be viewed on the Breastfeeding Report Card, published every two years:
• https://www.cdc.gov/breastfeeding/data/reportcard.htm

CHAPTER 1: PHYSIOLOGICAL HEALTH
Dose-related physical health benefits of breastfeeding or risks of not breastfeeding for mother and baby:
• https://www.ncbi.nlm.nih.gov/pmc/articles/PMC2812877/
• https://www.ncbi.nlm.nih.gov/pmc/articles/PMC6096620/
• https://onlinelibrary.wiley.com/doi/full/10.1111/mcn.12366

For data on the dose-related benefits of breastfeeding and the effects of increased breastfeeding rates on chronic disease reduction, see "Long-term effects of breastfeeding: A systematic review," written by Bernardo L. Horta, MD, PhD and Cesar G. Victora, MD, PhD and published by the World Health Organization in 2013:
• https://apps.who.int/iris/bitstream/handle/10665/79198/9789241505307_eng.pdf;
  jsessionid=791364D017943AE4603A468A0998777E?sequence=1

Information on metabolic disease:
• https://link.springer.com/article/10.1007/s11906-018-0812-z

Information on obesity and its relationship to mortality rates from the West Virginia Department of Health and Human Resources:
• www.wvdhhr.org/bph/oehp/obesity/mortality.htm

Information on breast cancer as it relates to lower breastfeeding rates:
"Breastfeeding and Breast Cancer Risk Reduction: Implications for Black Mothers" by Erica H. Anstey, PhD; Meredith L. Shoemaker, MPH; Chloe M. Barrera, MPH; Mary Elizabeth O'Neil, MPH; Ashley B. Verma, MPH; and Dawn M. Holman, MPH; published in the *American Journal of Preventive Medicine* in 2017:
• https://www.ncbi.nlm.nih.gov/pmc/articles/PMC6069526/

Information on diabetes risk reduction with breastfeeding, see "Lactation Duration and Progression to Diabetes in Women Across the Childbearing Years: The 30-Year CARDIA Study" by Erica P. Gunderson, PhD, MPH, MS; Cora E. Lewis, MD, MSPH; Ying Lin, MS; et al, 2018:
• jamanetwork.com/journals/jamainternalmedicine/article-abstract/2668634

The links below provide information on the specificity, bioactivity, and responsiveness of breast milk/breastfeeding:
• https://www.ncbi.nlm.nih.gov/pmc/articles/PMC3586783/
• https://www.ncbi.nlm.nih.gov/pmc/articles/PMC5005964/
• https://www.ncbi.nlm.nih.gov/books/NBK148970/
• https://www.ted.com/talks/katie_hinde_what_we_don_t_know_about_mother_s_milk/transcript?language=en
• http://humanmilkscience.org/Data/Sites/1/media/2017-conference/Proceedings_Keynote.pdf
• https://academic.oup.com/ajcn/article/110/3/769/5528418
• http://www.breastfeedingonline.com/HowBreastmilkProtectsNewborns.pdf

Milk Matters: Infant feeding & immune disorder, by Maureen Minchin (Milk Matters Pty Ltd, 2015): Medical historian and health educator Maureen Minchin has been involved in global efforts to promote evidence-based infant feeding for decades and is internationally recognized for her pivotal role in creating the lactation consultant profession. She has been a consultant to international bodies such as the WHO and UNICEF. She has educated health professionals, including through creating university-based courses in the UK and Australia, and is an Editorial Board member for the open-access online *International Breastfeeding Journal*. Learn more about *Milk Matters* at:
• https://infantfeedingmatters.com/milk-matters-the-book

Breastfeeding, New Anthropological Approaches, by Cecilia Tomori, Aunchalee E. L. Palmquist, and E.A. Quinn. Routledge, 2017.
• https://anthrolactology.com/about/
• https://anthropology.wustl.edu/people/ea-quinn

The CDC's diabetes report card and projections of diabetes incidence:
• https://www.cdc.gov/media/pressrel/2010/r101022.html
• https://www.cdc.gov/diabetes/pdfs/library/diabetesreportcard2017-508.pdf

For history and research on the importance of breastfeeding statistics, see:
• https://www.ncbi.nlm.nih.gov/books/NBK235588/
• https://www.acog.org/Clinical-Guidance-and-Publications/Committee-Opinions/Committee-on-Health-Care-for-Underserved-Women/The-Importance-of-Vital-Records-and-Statistics-for-the-Obstetrician-Gynecologist

The CDC's most recent Breastfeeding Report Card and our national breastfeeding goals:
• https://www.cdc.gov/breastfeeding/data/facts.html
• https://www.cdc.gov/breastfeeding/pdf/2016breastfeedingreportcard.pdf
• https://www.cdc.gov/breastfeeding/data/reportcard.htm

The CDC surveys on breastfeeding practices in the United States. Their National Immunization Survey (NIS) is used for estimates of vaccination coverage rates for US children aged 19 to 35 months. Since July 2001, breastfeeding questions have been asked on the NIS and are used to monitor breastfeeding rates at both national and state levels by birth year. All respondents (consisting of a random selection of 1% of each state's population) with children aged 19 to 35 months are asked four breastfeeding questions at the end of the long immunization survey. You can read about the survey:
• https://www.cdc.gov/breastfeeding/data/nis_data/index.htm

Information about how this survey is indicative of "trends" in breastfeeding rates rather than the concrete data that breastfeeding deserves:
• https://www.cdc.gov/breastfeeding/data/nis_data/survey_methods.htm

The Baby-Friendly Hospital Initiative is a plan and certification program to help hospitals give the best care to breastfeeding mothers and babies, reducing some of the barriers to breastfeeding within hospitals. Read more at:

• https://www.unicef.org/nutrition/files/BFHI_Case_Studies_FINAL.pdf

• https://www.babyfriendlyusa.org/for-facilities/practice-guidelines/10-steps-and-international-code/

The International Code of Marketing of Breast-milk Substitutes, aka "the Code," is a policy that the US has refused to enact. Additionally, the US has neglected to implement any policy or legislation to curb formula's inappropriate marketing practices. The following links discuss the Code and Conflict of Interest documents as they relate to formula marketing and its risks to breastfeeding success:

• http://www.who.int/nutrition/publications/code_english.pdf

• https://www.nytimes.com/2018/07/08/health/world-health-breastfeeding-ecuador-trump.html

• http://www.ncbi.nlm.nih.gov/pmc/articles/PMC2443254/

• http://www.washingtonpost.com/wp-dyn/content/article/2007/08/30/AR2007083002198.html

• https://www.unicef.org/nutrition/files/State_of_the_Code_by_Country_April2011.pdf

A recording of the 71st World Health Assembly (WHA) can be viewed online at

• https://www.who.int/world-health-assembly/seventy-first

The WHA's full discussion regarding the "Conflict of Interest" policy as it pertains to the marketing of breast milk substitutes can be read at

• http://apps.who.int/gb/ebwha/pdf_files/WHA71-A-B-PSR/A71_APSR11-en.pdf

Countries' representatives' remarks begin with Ecuador's comments on page 14 and end with the USA's on page 19. Note the USA's efforts to reduce protections against formula marketing via the promotion of "choice." Non-state actors' comments immediately follow the countries' comments, beginning on page 20.

The conflicts of interest at the 71st WHA are discussed in the "Report by the Director General to the 142nd Executive Board":

• https://www.who.int/nutrition/consultation-doi/comments/en/

Provisional agenda item 12.6 from the 71st WHA, titled "Maternal, infant and young child nutrition," can be read at

• http://apps.who.int/gb/ebwha/pdf_files/WHA71/A71_23-en.pdf

CHAPTER 2: DEVELOPMENTAL AND MENTAL HEALTH

To read more about the enhanced neurocognitive development of breastfed babies, see:

• https://www.thelancet.com/journals/langlo/article/PIIS2214-109X(18)30371-1/fulltext

• https://www.thelancet.com/journals/langlo/article/PIIS2214-109X(15)70002-1/fulltext

• http://www.ncbi.nlm.nih.gov/pmc/articles/PMC3916850/

• https://www.ncbi.nlm.nih.gov/pmc/articles/PMC6096620/

These articles contain information on the connections between breastfeeding, neurodevelopmental conditions, and mental illness:

• https://www.ncbi.nlm.nih.gov/pubmed/9246251

• https://www.ncbi.nlm.nih.gov/pmc/articles/PMC3981895/

• https://www.cdc.gov/ncbddd/autism/data.html

Find the Surgeon General's "Call to Action to Support Breastfeeding" and related information at:

• https://www.cdc.gov/breastfeeding/resources/calltoaction.htm

and find more information on how these actions are being implemented at:

• http://www.usbreastfeeding.org/action-directory

Recommendations regarding breastfeeding support in the US from the Surgeon General, CDC, and United States Lactation Consultant Association (USLCA) can be found at:

• https://www.surgeongeneral.gov/library/calls/breastfeeding/calltoactiontosupportbreastfeeding.pdf

• https://www.cdc.gov/breastfeeding/pdf/breastfeeding_interventions.pdf

• https://uslca.org/wp-content/uploads/2016/07/Efficacy-of-the-IBCLC.pdf

• https://www.dol.gov/whd/nursingmothers/faqBTNM.htm

• https://www.healthcare.gov/coverage/breast-feeding-benefits/

For numbers and staffing recommendations for IBCLCs and CLCs and information regarding certification, see:

• http://www.ilca.org/main/why-ibclc/ibclc

• https://iblce.org/about-iblce/current-statistics-on-worldwide-ibclcs/

• http://uslca.org/wp-content/uploads/2013/02/IBCLC_Staffing_Recommendations_July_2010.pdf

• https://nurse.org/education/certified-breastfeeding-lactation-councelor/

• https://www.cdc.gov/breastfeeding/pdf/2014breastfeedingreportcard.pdf

• https://www.liebertpub.com/doi/abs/10.1089/bfm.2016.0072?journalCode=bfm

• https://iblce.org/step-1-prepare-for-ibclc-certification/

• http://uslca.org/wp-content/uploads/2015/02/IBLCE-Stats-on-IBCLCs.pdf

• https://10301dl.com/wp-content/uploads/2019/04/Statistical-Report-IBCLCs-in-AMS-2019.pdf

NICU information on increased usage and overuse:

• https://pediatrics.aappublications.org/content/142/5/e20180457

• https://www.stltoday.com/lifestyles/health-med-fit/health/more-babies-going-to-the-nicu-and-more-than-half/article_03b339e0-0be1-5d99-ad38-9a17f54311e5.html

Postpartum depression (PPD) information:

• https://www.ncbi.nlm.nih.gov/pmc/articles/PMC4842365/

CHAPTER 3: GENDER, WORK, RACIAL, AND HEALTH EQUITY

Racial and geographic differences in breastfeeding rates:

• https://www.cdc.gov/mmwr/volumes/66/wr/mm6627a3.htm

"US support of formula over breastfeeding is a race issue":

• https://theconversation.com/u-s-support-of-formula-over-breastfeeding-is-a-race-issue-99987

• https://jamanetwork.com/journals/jamapediatrics/article-abstract/2748385

• https://www.cdc.gov/breastfeeding/pdf/breastfeeding-cdcs-work-508.pdf

• https://fns-prod.azureedge.net/sites/default/files/resource-files/FY2018-BFDLA-Report.pdf

Metabolic syndrome, pre-eclampsia, C-section rates, and maternal and infant mortality:

• https://www.ncbi.nlm.nih.gov/pmc/articles/PMC4516665/

• https://www.frontiersin.org/articles/10.3389/fendo.2017.00204/full

• https://www.preeclampsia.org/es/quienes-somos/53-health-information/532-preeclampsia-strikes-african-american-women-hard

• https://www.marchofdimes.org/Peristats/ViewSubtopic.aspx?reg=99&top=8&stop=355&lev=1&slev=1&obj=1

• https://www.hsph.harvard.edu/magazine/magazine_article/america-is-failing-its-black-mothers/

Black babies in the US die at just over two times the rate of White babies in the first year of their life, according to data from the US Centers for Disease Control and Prevention: for every 1,000 live births, 4.8 White infants die in the first year of life. For Black babies, that number is 11.7.

• https://www.cdc.gov/reproductivehealth/maternalinfanthealth/infantmortality.htm

• https://www.cdc.gov/nchs/pressroom/sosmap/infant_mortality_rates/infant_mortality.htm

To read about breastfeeding barriers in the US:

• https://www.ncbi.nlm.nih.gov/books/NBK52688/

To read more about fertility and birth rates in America, see:

• https://data.worldbank.org/indicator/SP.DYN.TFRT.IN?locations=US
• https://www.forbes.com/sites/ebauer/2018/09/26/
  will-the-fertility-rate-recover-probably-not-a-new-study-says/#3dc61af02268
• https://www.npr.org/sections/thetwo-way/2018/05/17/611898421/u-s-births-falls-to-30-year-low-sending-fertility-rate-
  to-a-record-low
• https://www.cdc.gov/nchs/data/nvsr/nvsr68/nvsr68_13-508.pdf
• https://www.thebalance.com/birth-rate-by-state-4684536
• https://www.census.gov/

Data regarding paid leave for families after the birth of a child or in times of illness can be found at:

• http://www.supportpaidleave.org/blog/
• https://www.motherjones.com/politics/2015/05/john-oliver-maternity-leave/
• https://www.ted.com/talks/jessica_shortall_how_america_fails_new_parents_and_their_babies
• https://effectivehealthcare.ahrq.gov/products/breastfeeding/research
• *Birth Strike: The Hidden Fight Over Women's Work*, by Jenny Brown, 2019. PM Press.

See analyses of breastfeeding-friendly policies, laws, paid leave, and work breaks at:

• http://www.who.int/bulletin/volumes/91/6/12-109363/en/
• http://breastfeedinglaw.com/
• http://www.ncsl.org/research/health/breastfeeding-state-laws.aspx
• https://www.dol.gov/whd/nursingmothers/

To read more in depth on the issues of working while breastfeeding, see the books *Breastfeeding and Employment: Making it Work*, Clinics in Human Lactation, Vol. 8, by Marsha Walker, RN, IBCLC, 2017, Praeclarus Press, and *The Big Letdown: How Medicine, Big Business, and Feminism Undermine Breastfeeding*, by Kimberly Seals Allers, 2017, St. Martin's Press.

The book *Breastfeeding, Social Justice, and Equity*, papers from the 10th Breastfeeding and Feminism International Conference in 2015, edited by Paige Hall Smith, Miriam Labbok, and Brittany D. Chambers, contains an in-depth analysis of the cultural, social, economic, and political influences of the American breastfeeding community.

CHAPTER 4: ECONOMIC HEALTH

To explore topics in breastfeeding and economics, GDP, poverty, and gender and equity issues, see the following:

- https://www.researchgate.net/publication/266382812_%27Lost_Milk%27-
- http://www.usbreastfeeding.org/dollars-sense
- http://www.nature.com/jp/journal/v22/n1/full/7210620a.html
- https://www.ncbi.nlm.nih.gov/pubmed/23855027
- http://www.peggyomara.com/2016/08/01/a-day-of-breastmilk-125/
- http://www.breastfeedingtas.org/about/economic_arguments_for_breastfeeding
- http://www.atlc.org/members/resources/JulieSmith/BFmeasure%20ECONOMIC%20%20P%2343B1A.pdf

- Margunn Bjørnholt and Ailsa McKay, "Counting Mothers' Milk in the United Nations' System of National Accounts—Progress in Principle," in *Counting on Marilyn Waring: New Advances in Feminist Economics* (Demeter Press, 2014):
- http://demeterpress.org/books/counting-on-marilyn-waring-new-advances-in-feminist-economics-second-edition/
- https://people.umass.edu/folbre/folbre/books.html
- https://slate.com/human-interest/2018/02/breast-milk-isnt-free.html
- https://www.ncbi.nlm.nih.gov/pubmed/11236730

- *The Big Letdown: How Medicine, Big Business, and Feminism Undermine Breastfeeding*, by Kimberly Seals Allers, 2017, St. Martin's Press.
- The conference paper "'Lost Milk?' – The Economic Value of Breastmilk in GDP," by Julie P. Smith, delivered in August 2014 at the ABA Liquid Gold conference in Melbourne, Australia.

For data on WIC costs and breastfeeding support and rates, see:

- https://www.cbpp.org/research/food-assistance/wics-competitive-bidding-process-for-infant-formula-is-highly-cost
- https://www.fns.usda.gov/wic/frequently-asked-questions-about-wic
- https://www.fns.usda.gov/wic/wic-breastfeeding-data-local-agency-report
- https://www.ncbi.nlm.nih.gov/pmc/articles/PMC1481608/
- https://www.fns.usda.gov/wic/breastfeeding-priority-wic-program
- https://www.fns.usda.gov/wic/legislative-history-breastfeeding-promotion-requirements-wic
- https://www.ncbi.nlm.nih.gov/books/NBK435907/#sec_000292
- https://s3.amazonaws.com/aws.upl/nwica.org/2018-wic-what-funding-basics.pdf
- https://www.ers.usda.gov/amber-waves/2004/september/
  sharing-the-economic-burden-who-pays-for-wics-infant-formula/
- https://www.ers.usda.gov/amber-waves/2019/february/economic-implications-of-increased-breastfeeding-rates-in-wic/
- https://fns-prod.azureedge.net/sites/default/files/ops/WICNSACostStudy.pdf

For information on infant formula, see: "Infant Formula: Evaluating the Safety of New Ingredients," Institute of Medicine (US) Committee on the Evaluation of the Addition of Ingredients New to Infant Formula, Washington, DC: National Academies Press (US), 2004:
- https://www.ncbi.nlm.nih.gov/books/NBK215837/
- https://babyformulaexpert.com/baby-formula-carbs/
- https://www.sciencedirect.com/topics/agricultural-and-biological-sciences/infant-formula

On the reduction of morbidity and mortality for mom and baby due to breastfeeding versus the risks of formula feeding and higher medical costs from not breastfeeding:
- http://flbreastfeeding.org/archiveFBC/HTMLobj-706/RisksofFormulaFeeding.pdf
- https://onlinelibrary.wiley.com/doi/full/10.1111/mcn.12366

To read more about the reduction of diabetes risk and costs from breastfeeding, see:
- https://www.nih.gov/news-events/nih-research-matters/
  breastfeeding-may-help-prevent-type-2-diabetes-after-gestational-diabetes
- https://jamanetwork.com/journals/jamainternalmedicine/article-abstract/2668634
- https://care.diabetesjournals.org/content/30/Supplement_2/S161
- https://www.niddk.nih.gov/health-information/health-statistics/diabetes-statistics
- https://care.diabetesjournals.org/content/early/2018/03/20/dci18-0007
- https://www.cdc.gov/diabetes/pdfs/data/statistics/national-diabetes-statistics-report.pdf

CHAPTER 5: ENVIRONMENTAL HEALTH
On the economic value of natural resources and why this should include breastfeeding:
- https://www.nap.edu/read/4844/chapter/2
- https://www.grin.com/document/283864
- http://i-tme.nl/pdf/assessment%20of%20econ%20value%20of%20environment%20final.pdf

On environmental issues and breastfeeding:
- http://www.who.int/mediacentre/commentaries/breastfeeding-in-emergencies/en/
- https://www.sciencealert.com/no-one-is-talking-about-the-environmental-impacts-of-the-baby-formula-industry

For information on breastfeeding and human milk research and need for funding:
- Katie Hinde, "What we don't know about mother's milk," TEDWomen 2016: https://www.ted.com/talks/
  katie_hinde_what_we_don_t_know_about_mother_s_milk
- https://www.ncbi.nlm.nih.gov/pmc/articles/PMC5005964/

- https://academic.oup.com/ajcn/article/110/3/769/5528448
- http://www.usbreastfeeding.org/p/cm/ld/fid=110
- http://www.midwife.org/nbrc-call-for-applicants

For information on milk banks and milk sharing, see:

- https://www.hmbana.org/
- https://www.google.com/maps/d/viewer?ll=40.64730399999999%2C-97.20703100000003&spn=31.887674%2C56.25&hl=en&t=m&msa=0&z=4&source=embed&ie=UTF8&mid=10fc70w_SGx2Bc_KQOzI2f_EPp0Y
- https://europeanmilkbanking.com/
- http://www.fiotec.fiocruz.br/en/news/4232-more-than-200-human-milk-banks-in-brazil-and-on-three-continents-network-celebrates-growth-and-success
- https://abm.memberclicks.net/assets/DOCUMENTS/ABM%27s%202017%20Position%20Statement%20on%20Informal%20Breast%20Milk%20Sharing%20for%20the%20Term%20Healthy%20Infant.pdf
- http://breastfeeding.sph.unc.edu/files/2014/11/DHM_I_Report_May-15-cost-truncated.pdf

CHAPTER 6: MATERNAL EMPOWERMENT

To read about the relation between breastfeeding, maternal empowerment, and self-sufficiency, see:

- http://www.marilynwaring.com/

For information about La Leche League, see:

- https://www.llli.org/about/
- www.llli.org/
- https://www.llli.org/about/history/

For information on the ratio of women versus men in the Nobel Prizes:

- http://stats.areppim.com/stats/stats_nobel_sexxcat.htm

For information on requesting a stamp from the United States Postal Service, see:

- https://about.usps.com/who-we-are/csac/welcome.htm
- https://about.usps.com/who-we-are/csac/process.htm

The following websites focus on breastfeeding art:

- http://www.fisheaters.com/marialactans.html
- https://www.theguardian.com/artanddesign/jonathanjonesblog/2014/dec/08/nigel-farage-breastfeeding-art-corner
- https://www.theguardian.com/artanddesign/jonathanjonesblog/2014/dec/08/nigel-farage-breastfeeding-art-corner

- https://www.amazon.com/Mother-Child-Commentaries-Distinguished-People/dp/B00002N71I
- https://www.instagram.com/breastfeedingart/
- https://www.pinterest.com/explore/breastfeeding-art/
- http://www.huffingtonpost.com/2015/05/19/breastfeeding-art-instagram_n_7314142.html
- https://www.pinterest.dk/pin/679973243710451892/
- https://19thcenturyrealism.com/category/gaston-parison/

CHAPTER 7: SOCIAL HEALTH

For more information about breastfeeding and working, see the book Breastfeeding and Employment: Making it Work, Clinics in Human Lactation, vol 8, by Marsha Walker, RN, IBCLC, 2017, Praeclarus Press, as well as the following:

- https://kellymom.com/hot-topics/milkproduction/
- https://www.bls.gov/news.release/pdf/famee.pdf
- https://www.womenshealth.gov/breastfeeding/breastfeeding-home-work-and-public/
  breastfeeding-and-going-back-work/business-case
- https://www.womenshealth.gov/files/documents/bcfb_business-case-for-breastfeeding-for-business-managers.pdf
- http://www.dol.gov/whd/nursingmothers/
- http://www.who.int/bulletin/volumes/91/6/12-109363/en/

To learn more about the various forms of breastfeeding legislation at state and federal levels, see the following:

- https://www.mamava.com/breastfeeding-laws
- http://www.ncsl.org/research/health/breastfeeding-state-laws.aspx
- http://revisor.mo.gov/main/OneSection.aspx?section=191.918&bid=9697&hl=breast-feeding%u2044
- https://health.mo.gov/living/families/wic/breastfeeding/resourcesdata/laws/
- https://en.wikipedia.org/wiki/Breastfeeding_in_public
- https://usbreastfeeding.salsalabs.org/2019pumpact/index.html?eType=EmailBlastContent&eId=eec
  0e155-bd2a-4be1-acb0-6fe648f970e6

MAP SOURCES:

WIC Breastfeeding Initiation Rates by State, 2018: U.S. Department of Agriculture, The Food and Nutrition Service, Special Supplemental Nutrition Program for Women, Infants, and Children. WIC Participant and Program Characteristics 2018 – Charts. Figure 4. Breastfeeding Initiation by State, 2004–2018. Accessed June 30, 2020. URL:

- https://www.fns.usda.gov/wic/participant-and-program-characteristics-2018-charts

US Initiation rates by state, 2016: Centers for Disease Control and Prevention. National Center for Chronic Disease Prevention and Health Promotion, Division of Nutrition, Physical Activity, and Obesity. Data, Trend and Maps [online]. [accessed June 25, 2020]. URL:
• https://www.cdc.gov/nccdphp/dnpao/data-trends-maps/index.html

Infant Mortality Rates by State, 2017: Centers for Disease Control and Prevention, Division of Reproductive Health, National Center for Chronic Disease Prevention and Health Promotion. Infant Mortality. Infant Mortality Rates by State, 2017. Page last reviewed: March 27, 2019. URL:
• https://www.cdc.gov/reproductivehealth/maternalinfanthealth/infantmortality.htm

Infant Mortality Rates by Race and Ethnicity, 2016: Centers for Disease Control and Prevention, Division of Reproductive Health, National Center for Chronic Disease Prevention and Health Promotion. Infant Mortality. Infant Mortality Rates by Race and Ethnicity, 2016. Page last reviewed: March 27, 2019. URL:
• https://www.cdc.gov/reproductivehealth/maternalinfanthealth/infantmortality.htm

Prevalence of obesity in the US in 2018: Centers for Disease Control and Prevention, Division of Nutrition, Physical Activity, and Obesity, National Center for Chronic Disease Prevention and Health Promotion. Adult Obesity Prevalence Maps. Map: Overall Obesity. Page last reviewed: October 29, 2019. URL:
• https://www.cdc.gov/obesity/data/prevalence-maps.html

County-Level Distribution of Diagnosed Diabetes Among US Adults Aged 20 or Older, 2013: Centers for Disease Control and Prevention. Diabetes Report Card 2017. Atlanta, GA: Centers for Disease Control and Prevention, US Dept of Health and Human Services; 2018.

Number and Percentage of U.S. Population with Diagnosed Diabetes, 1958–2015: Centers for Disease Control and Prevention, Division of Diabetes Translation, United States Diabetes Surveillance System. Long-term Trends in Diabetes, April 2017. Accessed Jun 30, 2020. URL:
• https://www.cdc.gov/Diabetes/statistics/slides/long_term_trends.pdf

Breast Cancer Mortality: U.S. Cancer Statistics Working Group. U.S. Cancer Statistics Data Visualizations Tool, based on 2019 submission data (1999-2017): U.S. Department of Health and Human Services, Centers for Disease Control and Prevention and National Cancer Institute; www.cdc.gov/cancer/dataviz, released in June 2020.

2017 Poverty Rate in the United States: United States Census Bureau, U.S. Department of Commerce, Economics and Statistics Administration. 2017 Poverty Rate in the United States. Last accessed: June 30, 2020. URL:
• https://www.census.gov/library/visualizations/2018/comm/acs-poverty-map.html

Find CDC maps of breastfeeding rates, illness rates, mortality, and poverty rates at:
• https://www.cdc.gov/breastfeeding/
• https://www.cdc.gov/breastfeeding/data/facts.html
• https://www.cdc.gov/obesity/data/databases.html
• https://www.cdc.gov/reproductivehealth/maternalinfanthealth/infantmortality.htm
• https://www.cdc.gov/diabetes/data/center/slides.html
• https://gis.cdc.gov/grasp/diabetes/DiabetesAtlas.html
• https://www.cdc.gov/diabetes/pdfs/library/diabetesreportcard2017-508.pdf
• https://www.cdc.gov/nchs/data-visualization/index.htm
• https://www.census.gov/library/visualizations/2016/comm/cb16-158_poverty_map.html
• https://www.cdc.gov/obesity/data/adult.html
• https://www.census.gov/library/visualizations/2016/comm/cb16-158_poverty_map.html

For diabetes information, see:
• https://diabeteswellbeing.com/diabetes-belt

About the Author

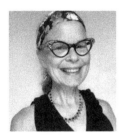 Erin L. O'Reilly is an RN, MSNR, IBCLC, volunteer La Leche League Leader, retired WIC Breastfeeding Coordinator, Public Health Nurse, Past President of the St. Louis Breastfeeding Coalition, and member of the Missouri Breastfeeding Coalition, the US Breastfeeding Coalition, the United States Lactation Consultant Association (USLCA), and the International Lactation Consultant Association (ILCA, ilca.org). She lives and works with the breastfeeding community in St. Louis, Missouri.

During her time as President of the St. Louis Breastfeeding Coalition, she helped to get a Missouri state breastfeeding law passed, obtain 501(c)(3) status for the coalition, and plan and fund the Breastfeeding Photo Project in 2014; helped write a grant for funding to start the I AM: Breastfeeding (breastfeeding) support group led by leaders in a Black community in St. Louis, which is still operating; as well as participated in many World Breastfeeding Week events over the years and other community events. She has been a volunteer La Leche League leader since 1999 and has led over 3,000 meetings as a Leader, taken countless phone calls, gone on many home visits to moms needing help with breastfeeding, and trained and certified many new La Leche League Leaders to continue the work of breastfeeding support. Erin taught childbirth and breastfeeding classes and worked in the lactation department of a major hospital in St. Louis for 19 years; she worked in the Nutrition and WIC Department in a neighborhood health care center as a Breastfeeding Coordinator from 2007 to 2020.

Erin's breastfeeding support experience has encompassed a wide variety of situations, and she has worked with many different women who have many different breastfeeding experiences, barriers, and/or supports. She breastfed her own son as well and experienced personally the barriers to breastfeeding, which inspired her to become a La Leche League Leader and an IBCLC to help others have an easier time on their breastfeeding journeys.

Contact Erin at ErinLOReilly.com.

CPSIA information can be obtained
at www.ICGtesting.com
Printed in the USA
LVHW071440090121
675817LV00002B/4

9 781734 438802